Raccoons Stole My Baby Jesus

Jennifer Doll, DVM

For Mom and Dad

Table of Contents

For Starters

"I feel the urge to fight all things practical." Jennifer Doll says to herself daily.

One important note: My mind wanders and my short term memory sucks. However, my long-term memory is incredibly vivid, and goes back to when I was two years old. A lot of people don't believe me, but it is true. Most of the memories are not of significant events, yet are so easy to recall that the colors and sounds and even smells come up if I let my mind wander. And man, .does my mind wander, like a pen scribbling on paper without stopping, going everywhere, and nowhere.

I have theories on why I have such a horrendous short term memory, yet an almost savant-like ability to recall the long ago past. It could be that when I was born my umbilical cord was wrapped around my neck for such a long time the family doctor, Dr. Mueller, told my mom that I was likely not to survive, and that if I did survive my birth I would be "mentally retarded."

Well, I'm not dead. Imagine how brilliant I could have been had I not been born mentally challenged.

I also blame frequent trauma to brain cells incurred during some incidents I may or may not remember to include in this book. For example: I was wrapped up by a 12-foot Burmese python while 5 months pregnant with my daughter Kirsten. I had a standoff with an adult male cougar armed with nothing but a ¾-inch long hypodermic needle. And, I went into DIC (definition to come) after being bit by a timber rattlesnake.

So if stories overlap... sorry about that. Welcome to my world.

Like any project, my life and profession has been a work in progress; hopefully progress is the key word. I was first a general small animal veterinary associate in Washington State; then owner of a mobile practice. Animals All About Inc., in Iowa; then founder and director of a shelter for special needs cats called Witty Kitties Inc.; and now medical director of Iowa Humane Alliance Veterinary Services Inc. Though my all-encompassing obsession with, and compassion for, animals started at the age of three, I'll skip the typical "I grew up on a farm and always loved animals...." schmaltzy, gushy, sweet story, even though it is true. My stereotypical interest in animals initially led to practicing as a veterinarian who did regular stuff and made decent money, until I moved to Iowa.

The fork in the road came along shortly after moving from Washington with my first husband. Until then I had been a veterinarian in private practice just outside of Seattle. The eight years there were spent in ignorant bliss, assuming among other things: all animals that went to shelters found homes; all shelters had money; and a veterinarian who loved taking care of shelter animals was paid well.

At that time I even had a *bad* impression of rescue groups, thanks to my initial exposure to one of them my first year out of vet school in 1991. A group I will simply call "Ego-Driven Animal Rescue" brought into the clinic a feral cat with a spinal injury. The cat was unable to walk, and was unable to empty her bladder. We call this an "upper neuron bladder," meaning the bladder fills and fills, but doesn't empty due to a spasm of the sphincter muscles. Only after it fills to a critical level will the cat empty just enough urine to release a little pressure. This results in repeated injury to the kidneys and stagnation of urine. Animals with this injury must have the bladder emptied manually, a difficult job with the tamest of cats. Unfortunately I was dealing with one of the most truly feral cats I would ever meet. ("Feral" is too often used for any stray or wildish cat.) This poor cat had to be netted multiple times a day to empty her bladder. When netting her, the poor thing first dragged herself in a panic in the cage, crawling with her front legs up the side. I shuddered to think of the damage being done to her already injured spine.

After two days of wrestling this panicked cat into a net, emptying her bladder, giving her antibiotics and fluids, I told the rescue I thought it best to put the cat down. I haven't even mentioned she had not eaten or drunk a bit the entire time she was with us. Boy, did I get an earful. "How can you be so cruel? You are a veterinarian. How could you suggest killing this innocent animal?" They picked up the cat the next day.

I found out the poor thing began having seizures two or three days later, and then died several hours after that. I don't doubt her kidneys had failed. She reportedly had been left in the cage and did not drink or eat the entire time.

It was then that I swore I would never EVER work with crazy animal rescue people.

I was wrong.

Ignorant Bliss

When Witty Kitties began so informally more than sixteen years ago, it was truly meant to provide a temporary shelter for a handful of kittens and cats I rescued when performing "mass neuters" at some rural Iowa farms.

Note: "Neuter" actually refers to the alteration of both male AND female animals to render them infertile. Because society seems to be afraid of saying "castrate" for male animals (as a companion to using "spay" for female animals), males seem to have claimed the word "neuter" as their own. I have been "corrected" by lay people for using the term for both males and females. "You **spay** females, not neuter." Thank you very much Dr. Layperson.

Anyway, the cats on these farms ranged from docile fat loaves that sat sunning on the porch all day waiting to be petted by anyone who cared to stop a moment, all the way to the absolutely crazy ones! I was forced to climb up onto rafters, on top of horse trailers and combines, stacked hay bales, and down into crawl spaces under sheds and even some kind of animal den on the side of a hill. You name it. My net and jab-stick (a three-foot pole I could attach a syringe full of sedatives into and use to inject an animal three feet away) were extensions of my arms on some of those days. I was scratched up so badly, not by cats, but usually by my surroundings. I suspect folks may have pegged me as a cutter.

What made it more difficult was having to get the cat into the veterinary van and provide an appropriately clean surgical environment in which to perform a spay or castration. My custom-built 24-foot-long veterinary vehicle had a separate surgery room, so I fortunately had a buffer zone in the non-surgery front portion of the van. Though providing mobile veterinary care was as complicated a practice as I could have imagined, I was determined to make it even more so.

It was the mid 1990s and my first husband, our son Joseph (aka JoJo), and I lived on a wooded 3-acre lot that shares a property line with the 14 acres where I currently live. My husband always liked animals, but was never insanely excited about them the way I was and am. He was wonderful at compromise and for that I am grateful. I had put my first rescued cats in our large screened porch, but was worried about the cold in the winter. He suggested appropriating our garage to create the cutest little cat shelter.

Darlene, my mobile clinic assistant, had a boyfriend, Kent, who built the first Witty Kitties shelter (before it had a name) in our two-car garage. It consisted of three rooms, each about 6 x 8 feet with high ceilings. The rooms were separated by clear Plexiglas to add to the light in all the rooms since I couldn't afford to add more windows in the garage. Kent was a perfectionist so everything was beautifully built. The woodwork was nicely stained, the quality doors to the rooms were well hung, and everything was square.

Though our marriage was coming to an end, my husband continued to compromise as best he could; but sometimes he had to be the "bad guy" when my desire to expand led me to bring home more and more animals. At the time it was thanks to him I wasn't already a hoarder. Again, I am grateful to him.

When I married my current husband, Torben, and moved onto the present 14 acres we own, things changed considerably. I no longer had someone who kept my drive to save animals in check. Torben has always been similar to me in his love and passion for animals, saying "yes" to anything that came our way.

When we bought the property, it included a crappy old farmhouse with no insulation in the upstairs rooms. I know this to be a fact thanks to peeking through a hole in JoJo's upstairs bedroom wall. I ended up expanding the hole and crawling into the wall in an attempt to replace the stupidly installed original insulation lengths. (Hey! It goes vertically between studs! Not stapled weakly from one end of the wall to the other!) I tell you this because I accidently stepped between the ceiling studs and fell through the living room ceiling. This is one of those rare fun stories that does NOT include an animal!

Torben and I moved the shelter to our "new" two car garage. This allowed us to make the three separate rooms much bigger, and include outdoor areas thanks to a large dog kennel attached to the back of the building. We were actually able to park a single car in it during perhaps the first 6 months we lived there. Torben and I intended to do nothing but continue with the cats, and to provide a huge yard for our dogs. The thousands of dollars in 4 foot high chain-link fencing was ALMOST perfect for the dogs. I say this because our border collie, Lucy, leaped over that sucker anytime she felt the need. The two strands of electric fence I then had to string down the length of the enclosure did nothing to stop her. This caused me so much distress because the road on which we live is a county road with a 55 mph speed limit. The ¼-mile stretch that is along our property line is a favorite racing spot. I don't have enough pages to write the names of all the dogs and cats from the neighborhood that have been killed along this road.

Lucy was such an odd dog, but very loving. She got really nervous with anything that was remotely violent and loud. If you swatted a fly in the house or even waved the fly swatter at something, she immediately got up, went outside, and jumped the fence. This in itself doesn't seem so weird. But what IS weird is that even if she was out in the yard and heard me swat a fly inside, she came in through the dog door to confirm it was indeed a flyswatter in my hand, and then ran out to jump the fence. Sadly, after a year Lucy managed to escape and was hit by a car. We found her body just inside a nearby horse pasture.

Despite its proximity to a busy road, we love our property. It is heavily wooded, with large meadows and rolling hills. It is beautiful place. Soon after we moved in, Torben and I decided to attend an exotic animal auction in a small Amish town south of where we live. At this time I was still very ignorant of the pitfalls of exotic animal breeding, as well as the rampant puppy mill business in that area. We went to see what "fun" animals we could see and perhaps even, gulp, buy. It is embarrassing to admit that we went to the auction to purchase animals. We were educated very early on in the trip as to the uglier side of the auction.

It was a very windy, cold April day. As we walked in, we had to go past an open building and were dismayed by the fact that people were selling iguanas and small pets from cardboard boxes and plastic containers in the outdoor area, despite temps being in the 40s. I couldn't believe the gall of the woman selling a darkened, stiff, cold iguana sitting on the bottom of a box. The owner claimed it sat so still because it was "tame." "More like soon to be dead," I thought. There were rabbits crowded into wire cages, sitting on top of each other, scared stiff. In the back of the building in the middle of an open area, sat several wire cages only about 1 ½ x 1 ½ x 1 foot, with adult foxes stuffed into them. I mean, they were completely exposed, no way to hide, and terrified. People just walked around them, poking them. Though completely wild and not handleable, the poor foxes were safe to touch because they couldn't even turn around in the pens! I was supremely saddened. Their eyes still haunt me.

It sickens me now to know I did not have the confidence in myself to speak out, to say that this was absolutely insane and cruel. It was all so shocking to me. My soapbox that today forces me to condemn this auction, that still continues every April and August each year, had yet to be built. So at the time, I said nothing, like a fool.

Torben and I continued to walk around in dismay, until we saw the llamas and emus. Suddenly we brightened. They absolutely fascinated us! The faces were the selling points on both counts. Llamas have big dark brown eyes with long lashes. Emus have this stare-you-in-the-eye-then-peck-your-eye-out look. The feathers on the tops of their heads looked like curly hair. They were wonderful; and with little thought as to why we shouldn't buy them or how we would get them home, we bought a llama, almost full-grown, two adult emus, and a baby goat.

It was only after the purchases were made when we thought, "Huh, how are we getting them all home?"

The town where the auction was held is almost an hour from where we live. What was our transportation? It was a VW van with a pop-up top. There were four of us: Torben, Joseph, a neighbor boy who tagged along on our adventures once in a while, and me. We decided to be "smart" and make two trips. The first trip home would be to deliver the boys, the goat, and the llama to our home. The guys at the auction house looked at us like we were insane, because we were. We had to wrestle Lorenzo the Llama (I had already named him) and plunk him into the back of the van through the hatch. If he kept his head down he could stand. I don't know how fondly Joseph thinks of that day, but I remember a lot of laughter from the boys at the time.

That trip wasn't too bad. We unloaded the two boys and two animals, letting the llama and goat run freely in our yard that circled the house, giving no mind to what neighbors just across the roads on two sides of our house would think, and headed back down to the auction barn. This time, when we backed the van up to the loading area, the guys, typical tough farm guys, asked Torben if we knew what we were doing. With a casual smile and a bit of machismo Torben replied, "Oh, yea. We've done this before." That was, sort of, ahem, a complete lie! Torben had seen Steve Irwin. the Crocodile Hunter, catch emus on television. Torben thought anything Steve could do, he could do.

Our van was backed up to the large barn doors which opened up to the long aisle that ran the length of the barn. On each side of the aisle were the pens. Torben and I just stood by the doors, waiting for the emus. We waited, excited, anticipating.

Way down at the other end of the barn a door on the right opened, letting out two emus. They stood for just a moment, looking at us, then ran straight for us. If you have never seen an emu, just imagine a slightly smaller ostrich. When they run, think of a velociraptor. When they kick, think of a kangaroo. Down the lane they came with their heads held low, level with their bodies, straight at us. I imagined some orchestra playing a march with pounding drums and shrill string instruments. Right at the door they stopped. They stood and looked around, and then Torben pounced down onto the back of one. Hugging it from behind, he took it to the back of the van as it kicked hard and fast at anything it could. Torben managed to get it into the van. I partially closed the hatch and watched as the other had to be cornered by the men who had been watching, wondering WTF they were seeing. Torben again grabbed this one from behind and took it to join the other in the van.

Torben looked at the guys and said "See ya" as though he was leaving a convenience store and had just purchased a soda. Eazy Peazy.

Our farm had been started. We were thrilled with our new pets, and thought it would all go spankingly after that. The emus did what they do, ran up and down and up and down the long length of fence that parallels the racetrack of a road along it. Lorenzo was aloof, yet happy to meet up with us when we had food. After a quick education on the needs of goats, llamas, and emus (and purchasing the proper foods), we felt fully competent.

Until both emus jumped the fence.

Evidently most emus will stay in confines with fences only 3 feet high IF they are in a group they are attached to. The male and female emus we had purchased came from different groups (welcome to the world of exotic pet sales). They didn't know each other and certainly didn't know our place as home. Seems when an emu is running fast, like the prehistoric-looking thing it is, it can then hook a foot onto the fence and hop right over. We had been warned at the barn about this, but we were in stupid animal-buyer mode at the time.

I was at work in the back of my Animals All About mobile van doing surgery when I got a call from our friends that the emus were at large. Torben was at his job as Director of a local Humane Society when the call came. He was able to get some help and go hunt down the one that had been sited last. Before heading out he spoke with an emu farmer on how to catch an escaped emu. What was the best way to do it?

"You don't," Was the reply. "You shoot' em."

Well that seemed extreme.

Torben rallied our friends. Some of this is a blur, so we'll just say a small army was gathered. They cornered one emu on a road that dead-ends into a local lake and jumped on it. This time the emu went absolutely berserk and kicked like hell. Torben was not going to be able to hold it and carry it to the vehicle. Someone took off his belt and wrapped the bent legs up against the body. The army then carried the bird back to the van and drove it home. I think this was the last day we ever had a vehicle in our garage because they put the emu into it.

The other emu, the male, was still at large. I was worried not only for its safety but for the safety of people should the emu race into traffic. It must have been 4 or 5 days later when I was driving my van home from a work day. Joseph and his friend, who were about 6 years old at the time, were riding in the back. I don't really remember why. We were on the winding part of the road that straightens out as it runs past my house, less than half a mile from home, when I saw two people standing in a front yard looking at....an emu! I slammed on the brakes and turned into the driveway and parked. There was an older boy, and a man (who I may or may not have met more than once before this but who is now a dear friend) standing about twenty yards from the emu.

I don't remember much about discussing a catch plan. I think I behaved as though I had done this before. Guess I'm a quick study to my teacher Torben. Sure wish I had the others' point of view on how well that was carried out! I got only a few feet from our emu, which surprised me. It must have been tired of running I guess. I then heroically leaped on it. I, the first man, and a third man (who was another neighbor and future friend) carried it with its head covered (by a sock?) to the van. They followed me home to help move the emu. After parking, I opened the door of the van and saw a still body. The emu had died. This susceptibility to dying under stress is something I had read about after the day they escaped.

It saddened me that we had failed our emus.

We then had to face the fact that we had a single emu, which wasn't optimal.   (Ideally, emus live in groups or pairs.) So off we went to an emu farmer who lives several miles north of Cedar Rapids. While there, we interrogated him on other emu oddities such as: If you introduce an emu's babies to it after hatching them in an incubator they will kill it. If they don't recognize a much smaller animal that does not look like another adult emu they will stomp them. I have come to witness that; but that is another story. We paid some money and put the new, young adult, emu in, no, not the VW van. We had driven my Saturn station wagon. We had put the back seats down and forced that bird into the far back. Yep, just another Sunday drive with Mom and son in the front and Dad in the back. Popping up over the back seat in the rearview mirror, the family emu's head bobbed about, looking around inquisitively.

That was the last time we actively looked for and bought a pet until 14 years later when we acquired a guinea pig for our daughter.

All future animals would NEED us: caimans, alligators, pythons, raccoons, bears. We would take them all

Maybe it's Maybelline…

Each year a popular veterinary journal has a contest called "They Ate WHAT?!" which draws in veterinarians all over the world to show off radiographs of dogs, cats, even toads who had ingested objects too large to be believed. Actual swallowed objects include steak knives; huge quantities of rock; toys that appear almost as big as the head of the animal who had eaten them (I'm not talking snakes here); even pet cats, collars and all (I AM talking snakes here). Some are incredibly cool, and some awfully sad, but the contest is always something I look forward to each year.

Though I've taken some fun things out of bellies, such as bras, a hard plastic Incredible Hulk hand, and game pieces, I have no idea how to categorize the case in which I had to remove an object from another portion of the body.

This happened in about 2002. Torben was still the director of a Humane Society where I would spend a day each week examining animals and neutering them in my van. Clara Belle (or something like that) was an approximately 3 year old basset hound who had been running at large. After the 7 day waiting period no one had come to claim her so she was put onto my list of patients. Clara Belle's spay was uneventful despite her being in-heat. It is pretty common to see in-heat dogs show up at shelters because their hormones lead them astray, looking for love like one of those girls we always seem to know who gets totally smashed at the bar every time you go out, then leaves you alone to go home with a new guy. Not that that has ever happened to me. Ok, I was often a third wheel.

But anyway... Clara Belle had an approved adoption application at the time I spayed her. So the day after surgery the happy family picked her up. A week later I was told the new owner was concerned about discharge coming from her "you-know-what"."That is what she said. As a joke I wanted to say "What What?" but am always the professional. Knowing what she meant I said, "Her vagina?" Yes, her vagina still had a bloody discharge. I explained this is common for dogs spayed while in pre or early heat and that it should diminish as time goes on.

A week later, Clara Belle was scheduled to meet me at the shelter because now, not only did Clara Belle have an increasing discharge, it was getting.......rotten smelling.

OK, the dog was running around happy. She had no fever. The microscope sample showed a bad vaginal infection. I put her on antibiotics.

A week later Clara Belle was back and the owner, who wasn't angry, really wanted to know what to do. Looking at that big sagging face, her mouth open and panting, tail wagging, I just thought "WTF Clara Belle? Whatcha been doin' back there?"

I anesthetized Clara Belle. A vaginal exam revealed nothing. Worried I had an infection at the site where the portion of the uterus was removed, I opened her belly. I saw nothing out the ordinary. What could possibly be going on? Her urine was normal. Check. Her uterine stump was normal. Check. The vagina was normal, except for having the discharge coming from upstream. Check. So I had a problem in a portion of the reproductive tract that we vets usually don't see when spaying a dog since there is no real reason to. It is from the cervix, and down. This area is hidden by the pubic bone. (Just think of that bone you hit when falling onto the bar of a girl's bicycle.)

Cutting the bone was not at the top of my options list, a tad extreme. So there I was, standing looking into Clara Belle's open belly, in the back room of my van, facing a dilemma I had to deal with on my own. It was at these times I missed working with other doctors, and having a sounding board to bounce my ideas off. I wanted to ask someone how to explore this "black box" inside this dog without an endoscope that I could just pass up there and look. I am sure at the time I was indeed talking to myself out loud, which I am known to do. After going over the list of options to myself, I figured out a productive solution.

I decided to keep my right hand sterile and inside Clara Belle's belly, then contaminate my left hand and insert my fingers into her vagina. I then pushed down hard on her uterine stump with my right hand......and there it was. With just the tip of my finger of my left hand I felt something solid, very hard. Unfortunately it was difficult performing this technique which I call the "pectoral curl with a twist." I called Torben to come out of the shelter, clean up, and don surgical gloves.

So as a lovely husband-wife team, Torben pushed down on Clara Belle's innards and I grasped desperately at an object which was very slippery and seemed long. I finally was able to safely grab it with a forceps and pull it out. Ta da! Mystery solved! What I found to be in Clara Belle was completely unexpected.

It was a Maybelline mascara tube. Now at first the object's identity wasn't obvious to me because, as you can imagine, being in a dog's hooha for several weeks did a lot to disguise it. It had a nasty black film over it. Once cleaned, I found it to be the brand I had used in high school, back in the early 80s when all girls wore black eyeliner on both lids and tons of mascara. It was the pink tube with a green cap. I was excited to tell the owner I finally had an answer to Clara Belle's problem and that she should be good to go after another week of antibiotics for residual infection. It gave me great satisfaction to show her the culprit, and I half expected her to be so excited that she would want to take the mascara home to show people as well. You know, like keep it on the shelf so when company came over she could start a conversation like, "You'll never guess where that came from." Or she could include it in a game, like "what is pink and green and lives in the dark?" But the owner, though grateful, did not need the mascara, and I think was feeling weird about having to explain to the rest of her family, if at all.

For me, I was proud, and actually saved that stupid thing in a sealed plastic bag for many years. After finding it in my basement in a box of miscellaneous vet stuff I hadn't been using, I looked at it one more time (without opening the bag), then tossed it out. But I never could use that brand again, though I know it is still available. I can't say I've ever gone into a make-up aisle at the store and NOT thought of Clara Belle every time I see the mascara shelves. My eyes always look around for the pink and green container, like a compulsion. I like to think of how much better Clara Belle felt after having the object removed, though her mood had always been happy-go-lucky every time I saw her.

I have decided not to elaborate further on my theories on just HOW a container of mascara ended up in Clara Belle, since I feel I've grossed you out with my descriptive terms, like vagina, uterine stump, and hooha. I leave that to your imagination. I try not to think about it.

Heart Breakers

Dealing with animals day in and day out, especially those that hadn't had homes prior to coming me, is a very rewarding endeavor. If it weren't for those moments of joy when an ill animal is finally feeling better, or a once stray cat finds a loving home, or a shelter cat purrs while curled up in your lap, NO one could stay in the animal rescue "business" for long.

However, for every joyous event, there are at least as many heartbreaking stories. Since we lost our first witty kitty, Jasper, in 2000, to feline leukemia virus-related problems, we have had dozens of kitties come and go in our lives, each one leaving his or her own paw prints on our hearts.

I remember Scamper, who came in 2001. He was a young adult, black domestic short hair who had been paralyzed in his back legs, but had slowly gained the ability to stand on his hocks (ankles) and even step. Because the back of the lower part of the leg isn't well protected by leathery pads like the bottom of the paws, the skin between his feet and ankles eventually developed deep wounds from rubbing. By the time I met him he had exposed bone and infection at the site of the sores. He was also fecal incontinent so would sometimes soil that portion of his legs. To help protect his legs I made him "orthopedic shoes," which were simply leg splints that I wrapped on the outer side of his legs. With these he could stand upright, and even walk, though very straight-legged as the splints extended just above the knees.

Scamper was very active once he got his special legs. He would run stiff-legged in my yard which was a real treat since he was otherwise caged. He would make his way to his favorite cedar tree where he would sit back on his rump, legs straight in front of him, and stare up at birds he would never be able to catch. Because of the fecal soiling, the wraps on the splints had to be changed almost daily. Faced with this and the ever-open sores, the partial paralysis on his back half, and his little "orthopedic" shoes to protect his legs from getting sores, I considered fusing his ankles. We just needed to clear up the infection before doing so. It was really a bit of a vicious circle of circumstances.

At the time we didn't have the army of volunteers Witty Kitties enjoys now. So much of my time was spent cleaning the shelter as well as performing all veterinary duties. The combination of the time it took caring for Scamper, trying to keep Lucy in the yard, and fixing the fence (where Lorenzo the Llama leaned against it bending the top bar, or where the goat had managed to rub against it and stretch it to the point that animals could crawl under it – chain link fencing is not optimal for farm animals!) was tough on me and my family. At the time, I didn't have relationships with people who could help foster Scamper, unwrap and rewrap his splints, or even tell me whether putting so much effort into a single cat outweighed how much help I could give to less disabled cats, or time I could spend with my family.

I cried as I put Scamper down, apologizing to him for not being a better, stronger person. To this day, more than 15 years later, his "shoes" still hang in the Witty Kitties infirmary room. They automatically bring the image of him sitting under that tree, staring straight up at the birds. He sat warmed by the sun, not knowing that that was the best it was ever going to get.

Another witty kitty who left an indelible mark in my memory was Mike. There was a time when I couldn't scoop litter boxes in one of our feline leukemia virus (FeLV) rooms without having the eerie feeling that Mike, a very large, black and white tuxedo domestic short hair, was going to sneak up behind me and jump up on my back if I was leaning over, or my shoulders if standing up. To counteract any negative feelings I may have had toward him due to this habit, Mike made sure to make me laugh as well. If I bounced a ping pong ball he would catch it, then stuff it in his mouth and carry it around. He could do so without needing to dent the ball at all. It was hilarious. Sadly the memory leads inevitably to having to put him down due to FeLV-related pneumonia. He was such a character and sometimes a pain in the butt, making my heart always skip a beat when he'd first land on me. The animals with the biggest personalities leave the biggest void once they are gone.

I could go on forever with stories, but I have to say the kitty that won over the most hearts during her time here was Peanut.

Peanut came to us in March of 2003. She was brought to us by a young woman who had been renting a house in the country, and had become friendly with the local farm cats. Two years prior, she took in a tiny kitten that had been injured. The kitten was suffering from a dislocated right shoulder and jaw. A veterinarian was able to replace the shoulder, but didn't observe the jaw problem at the time. Soon after, the jaw fused in its dislocated almost-closed position. The kitten, named Peanut, couldn't open her mouth. Her good Samaritan fed her especially mushy food which Peanut was able to suck through her teeth. This kept her going, but she was constantly hungry, as she could never fill herself up.

Even with all the old food and drool on her face, chest, and front legs (despite frequent cleaning by her rescuer), and her general stinkiness, Peanut looked like a happy, healthy (though thin) cat when she arrived at Witty Kitties. We took her in and fed her in the manner to which she'd been accustomed, three times daily. It wasn't long before I decided to put her under anesthesia to get a good look at her mouth. I discovered the lower jaw had dislocated, and was displaced caudally (towards the back), and tilted. Her teeth were all overlapping, and only had the tiniest spaces through which to suck her food. After giving her a ton of preemptive pain killers, I removed all the teeth I could with the little exposure I had. Due to the tilting of the lower jaw, some had to be removed by taking out a bit of bone. A few hours after surgery, to my surprise, Peanut was half awake and purring! I can still see her as she groomed herself for the first time since she was a young kitten. She could get her tongue out of her mouth! She wasn't the prettiest sight at that moment, due to the blood and drool she was spreading over her body. But boy *was* she happy!

Peanut could finally lap up food, and she was able to fill her belly with as much as she wanted at a sitting. This allowed us to only have to feed her twice daily. We fed her canned food, supplemented with milk replacer. Soon she was carrying surplus weight, and seemed proud of it. Peanut initially lived in our old shelter (the garage). Then we allowed her to live in our home for several months. I admit, though it was not a "love-hate" relationship we had, it was something like an "I-love-you-but-don't-get-so-close-to-me" relationship. Peanut still drooled and accumulated a lot of food on her face when she ate. We were constantly wiping her face, and the area around her dish. She tended to smell bad, despite regular bathing. This was a problem, as she was a very loving kitty, enjoying a lap to sit on, and rewarding you with nuzzling to your face.

Many nights we woke to see her funny, tongue-sticking-out face staring down at us, blowing bad breath on us, and kissing us. Though she could pull her tongue completely inside her mouth if she wanted, she rarely did. She liked to let it hang out, and due to her undershot jaw, it REALLY hung out there. She was messy and added to the already numerous chores in the house, so, after finding out I was pregnant with Kirsten, we moved her to our new larger shelter that had just been completed. Her room was like a small living room with a couch, trees, and a cat door going to an outdoor enclosure where she could climb onto shelves high above our heads.

Peanut wasn't happy about her new home at first, but soon was discovered by visitors and volunteers who took pity on her and gave her the attention she craved. When folks came to our shelter, Peanut was often the first kitty they saw as her outdoor enclosure was at the front of the building. Her dirty and dry tongue was cause for amusement in some, and dismay in others. "Why don't you amputate that?" Believe me, I heard that more than once. We continued giving her the special food mixture and cleaning up the big mess afterwards. Peanut was truly the epitome of the "special needs" kitty.

Ten months later, I was surprised one evening to find a large amount of blood in her dish. I briefly looked at Peanut's tongue, figured she must have gotten a scratch on it, as it was so prominent, and let it be for the night, expecting it to be no big deal. Next day, the same thing happened. There was so much fresh blood in her dish I decided to anesthetize her so I could do as thorough an exam as possible. I examined as much of her tongue and mouth as I could see, which wasn't much, and let her wake up. The scene replayed itself the next day as well: blood, anesthesia, nothing, wake up.

The entire time this was happening, Peanut appeared to feel fine. She had no idea she had a problem. I brainstormed on breaking her jaw, to allow a better view of her mouth and throat. I considered finding a vet with a fiber optic scope that was only a few millimeters in diameter. Once again, I wondered, "How far do I go?" This is a dilemma many owners face with their pets, and I'd faced many times before. We were concerned about the amount of pain she would need to endure with surgical exploration of the area. I needed to find if the blood was coming from her throat or esophagus, and why. But once I knew, then what? We also have the sad fact that money and time must be spread over several dozen cats. An MRI or CT scan was out of the question. "The need of the many outweighs the need of the few" is a frequent saying at many shelters.

In the end, we decided that we should euthanize Peanut while she still felt good, for it is a rule at Witty Kitties that no one suffers. After putting Peanut down, and crying a tremendous amount, I made myself take a look at Peanut's mouth and throat. It was a difficult task and I won't go into details. As it turned out, she had a mass in her pharynx. During earlier exams I hadn't seen many polyps and I knew they are benign; but to remove everything would have been impossible without intensive surgery to her neck and throat.

Peanut is buried under a tree near the shelter, and continues to pop into my mind when I walk past her. I like to remember how funny she looked, and how happy she always seemed with herself as she would rub her drool-soiled face against mine in the morning. I have a favorite photo of Peanut that was taken by a wonderful volunteer and friend of ours and Witty Kitties. It is of Peanut sitting in the driveway, staring at a mouse she or another cat had caught. She looks content, though there is no way she could ever eat that mouse. Images like that, and Peanut's joyful, yet short time here keep me going. It's why I keep doing what I can to make even the tiniest moments as wonderful as possible for all the witty kitties.

Should I Follow My Head? Or My Heart? .....Or My Gut? (The story of Sid and Rip)

This is so typical:

One day I was getting towards the end of a day of work at one of the local shelters. My mind was on my work most of the time, but kept returning to a particular cat I had met earlier in the day. I guess you could say I was even a bit obsessed at times, finding myself more distracted by him as the day wore on. This isn't unusual for me.

This cat was like thousands I'd met before. He was homeless. There was nothing new there. Mind you, I often am consciously trying to put the local unwanted pet population problem in perspective as it relates to all the human and animal suffering that goes on around the world. I remind myself how lucky I am to be who I am, where I am, in the time I am. So why couldn't I ignore this one cat and get on with my work? He was a stray cat. That wasn't my fault. Humans have inflicted domestication and homelessness on cats for so long. I am just one person.

But.... when the problem is in close proximity to me, the need to do something immediately is quite demanding. I actually was feeling I "owed" it to this cat more than most.

Why? I've seen hundreds of cats who would never find homes, who would be euthanized for lack of space and money for shelters. As a vet, I had been learning to take part in that difficult dynamic, comforted only by the knowledge that if I could help a cat die with as little mental and physical pain as possible, I would be giving him a passing that would otherwise not have been so peaceful.

What was so special about this cat? Well, when the Humane Society staff picked him up, he was extraordinarily thin and dehydrated, eyes sunken, and coat tragically unkempt.

So what? So many strays came this way. One difference was he also suffered from a severe dislocation of the left knee. From the feel of it, it had been like that long enough for the muscle and other soft tissue to not permit easy replacement. At any rate, he couldn't stand on it.

So what? Cats came in frequently with similar injuries, and we shouldn't be surprised by that. Well, since this cat was unable to lie on his left side, he had been hunkering down in the horrendously cold weather for the last few weeks, lying primarily on his right side. Thanks to the super sub-zero temps of the last week, he developed frostbite to both right paws, which were swollen to the size of baseball mitts. If it were not so sad, I'd have laughed at how funny they looked when I first saw him. I mean they were huge.

So what? We were seeing tons of cats with frostbite that time of year. But (and this was a big "but"), this cat was a four-paw declaw, meaning all four paws were without nails. To make it worse, his only good leg wasn't "good" either! The left foreleg, the one that wasn't frostbitten and didn't have a dislocation, had a re-growth of the nails. This happens when a tiny piece of the bone that is removed when a toe is declawed is accidentally left behind during surgery. As the new nail grows from the left-behind bone, it breaks its way through the skin. To say the least, this is painful and almost always ends in a stinky infection.

Soapbox time: I hate declawing. I used to declaw cats. For 8 years right out of school, I did the surgery because we were taught that is was a way to make cats more appealing to owners, and would help cats get or keep homes. Not once was a negative consequence mentioned in regards to the procedure. Now, after years of NOT performing declaws, I can guarantee you there are many behavioral and physical problems associated with declawing that occur in at least a third of declawed cats within 3 years of the procedure.

Declawing removes the last bone of the toe, not just the claw. When this is done, the next bone up on the toe curls downwards, leading to walking on the tip of the bone which is just under the pad and is often damaged after the procedure. Cats compensate by tilting their "wrists" back, and often develop arthritis higher up on the leg. This chronic pain can lead to cats not using the litter box. Also, cats who can't warn you not to pet them learn to bite. Even the CDC recognizes this and states declawing should not be performed on a cat in a household with an immunosuppressed person.

I can go on and on (needn't be such a bummer right now). But if you are one of the few lucky people who got away with declawing your cat and have not had to witness any of the complications, it doesn't make it OK. Oh, and give it time. Behavioral issues due to pain can manifest years after declawing.

The Humane Society checked for a microchip, and traced the cat back to his owner. His owner, who had adopted the cat from a shelter two years prior, wasted no timehaving the cat declawed on all four paws, making the cat almost defenseless. Then he allowed the cat to go outside. His owner never looked for him to bring him in from the cold and, when notified that his cat had been found, he wasn't interested in him. Even worse, the shelter was currently filled to capacity with healthy cats -- cats that would find homes without the shelter spending a tremendous amount of money it didn't have anyway. It wasn't looking good for this poor boy. Despite all of his problems, he nibbled on his food, and made himself comfortable in his box. I had no way of knowing for sure just how accustomed he was to whatever amount of pain he was in, but he did seem content with just being warm and secure.

After checking him out that morning I went back to my usual work, trying to forget his likely fate. I reminded myself of all the other cats who could be helped with less effort. Maybe he was suffering to the point where helping him wasn't really helping him. The question "Is it worth it?" is familiar to vets and pet owners alike in such cases.

I was troubled, asking myself "Should I follow my head?" This would be my logical brain that looks at only the practicality and logistics of a situation. "My heart?" My heart is all about what I want and uses the emotions that come to the surface during a situation. "My gut?" Many may say one's heart and gut are one in the same. But I disagree. I feel my gut is the intuitive part of me. I can't really explain it, but it is just what it sounds like, guttural. It tends to be the tie-breaker between decisions being pondered by my heart and head. I won't say which I listened to, but it was a vote of two-to-one. I took the majority. I gave in.

His name was Sid. Once I got Sid home, I found he was even worse off than I thought. I had tried giving him antibiotics for his infected toe and soon-to-slough skin from the frostbite. But getting pills down his throat was very difficult. I just couldn't get his jaw open wider than about 2 cm. After a few tries, I switched to liquid. Though his jaw felt normal and was symmetrical, I could only assume he had some sort of damage to the joints of his jaw. I'd missed this earlier because it didn't hinder his eating whatsoever.

Two days later Sid became even more interesting. While under anesthesia, I found he certainly didn't have the mechanical ability to open his jaw any wider. I debrided (removed) some of the tissue that was sloughing from the three paws. I decided not to cut back on his pain meds. I still didn't address the dislocation as it had been like that for a long time. Healing from the more acute injuries and getting stronger was more important at this point.

Eventually, as he healed, I had to make a decision about the knee dislocation. As it turned out, he had a fracture at the end of his femur (thigh) bone, near the knee. The result was that the small broken piece and the rest of the knee were positioned way up in his groin. Even if I could manage to get everything back into place to fuse the knee, it would have meant more weeks of pain, metal implants, more open wounds . . . So I decided to salvage the situation and amputate the leg. In just a matter of days, his "leg" would feel fine. He hadn't been able to use it anyway, so he would get used to the change more quickly than most. Oh, I ALSO had to remove the remaining piece of bone that was growing the nail that had punctured through his skin as a result of the declawing.

So, after several more days of pain medication and injectable antibiotics, he was moving around and gaining weight and strength. While checking on him morning and night, it never ceased to amaze me when he'd show me those bright eyes he had not been able to show on the first day. The two-to-one vote between my head, heart, and gut was a success, and very soon Sid became a beloved indoor pet.

You'd think cats as bad off as Sid don't come along too often, but only four days later, at another shelter, I came across a similar, but less dramatic, "add insult to injury" situation. I named him Rip. As in "to tear" (not as in "Rest In Peace") or as in Rip Torn, the comedian. You'll see why.

Rip walked into a person's yard a few days earlier dragging a leg-hold trap on one of his front legs. (*Future soapbox: Leg-hold traps should be illegal!*) Fortunately for Rip, the folks who found him were able to remove the trap and called friends who brought him to the shelter. He wasn't extremely thin, so I assumed he had someone feeding him at some point. But after the requisite waiting period for strays, an owner never showed up.

The shelter wasn't ignoring his paw. They were giving him antibiotics, and had given him the routine vaccinations all incoming cats get. But he was going to lose all the skin on a few toes, leaving his paw essentially skinned (like those poor animals the leg-hold traps were meant for). He would eventually need to have them amputated. This was something the shelter may not be able to afford, especially given the overcrowded conditions. As an injured and unneutered cat, Rip wouldn't be next in line for the adoption room. No, the adoption room was also filled to capacity.

Next in line for the adoption room were a half dozen healthy, beautiful, and already neutered adult cats waiting for a spot to open as soon as an adoption was made. Also in line were other healthy and beautiful cats who still needed neutering but had no other issues. And then there were the not-so-healthy, yet fairly comfortable and easily treatable sick or hurt cats. Then we get to where Rip sat. If Rip were a kitten, he may have the chance to "butt" in line ahead of the others, but he was about a year old. Granted, he was sweet, very tame, and cute, just not "kitten cute."

So, what happened to Rip? He ended up being a win/win situation after all. At the end of my work day, I "quickly" sedated him, tested him for feline immunodeficiency virus and feline leukemia virus, neutered him, and amputated the toes of the bad paw, all on my own time. I really did not have room at my home and Witty Kitties had its own waiting list, so I just asked that the shelter try putting him up for adoption. Though full of cats, the shelter felt he was sweet enough that he should find a home. Heck, some people actually want a handicapped pet. A mildly gimpy cat was going to sell himself. And so he did, quickly right into a home.

Time and time again I toil with problems like this. Shelter and rescue folks try to weed through who can be treated, who is most adoptable, who is suffering too much to even attempt treatment. I am always asking if it is a hero complex that makes me want to take on these odd cases. Or is it guilt, because we humans have insulted or mistreated them in so many painful ways? Is it reasonable to do the objective thing, and follow my head? "Follow logic and reason, Jenni!" But the heart says, "No! Do the 'kind' thing!"

It is at the point when my head and heart are in most disagreement that my gut comes in to break the tie. I admit I don't always listen to the majority vote, and often end up flying by the seat of my pants, hoping for the best outcome for all involved, especially the animals. Sadly, there are simply no easy answers in this constant struggle between head, heart, and gut.

Blind Leading the Blind: Lions, Tigers, and Bears! (Without the Tigers)

The recent presidential election (talking 2016 here) has had a lot of us slack-jawed and disbelieving. I am personally asking myself when was the last time I thought I was living in a totally crazy world, where "yes" meant "no" and "down" was "up". Believe it or not, I have an answer to that. I refer to an experience during a specific three weeks of my life from mid-July to early August of 2006. During that time I had multiple opportunities to think to myself, "What the heck am I doing? This can't be happening! When will I learn that this doesn't make sense!?"

Let me start with the "It'll-never-happen-again-in-my-lifetime" situation: Picture if you will a reluctant veterinarian riding as a passenger in the cab of a big diesel pickup. In the open back of the pickup were four large plastic dog crates, each containing an adult cougar that had just been removed from a neglect situation. All were under some level of sedation that the veterinarian had provided earlier. The truck was towing a very large horse trailer containing a half-asleep adult black bear.

Now, for those of you who know about big cats, you can imagine plastic dog crates are **not** optimal, as the cats can break out easily if awake. The reluctant vet had **no** part in the decision as to how these cats would be transported.   Her vet services were needed to sedate the animals for the ride to new, temporary homes.

Little did anyone know at the time, but each crate was missing at least one bolt that holds the top and bottom together. And little did they know, either, that the one crate missing a bolt on **both** sides, nearest the crate door, contained the least sedated cougar, the big male.

Okay, by now you know I am the reluctant veterinarian in the passenger seat. Why reluctant? Well, though I was eager to help when I got the desperate phone call about the poor conditions these animals were living in, I did **not** want anyone thinking I had experience with these animals. Truth is, I had **never** touched an adult cougar, let alone sedated one for transport. Unfortunately, when I said I was willing to help, it translated into "She's the vet who is going to take care of these animals, including figure out where they will go once removed from the property."

Anyway, the driver and owner of the pickup truck was a very mild-mannered man I'll call Danny. He had volunteered to be the driver as he often did for an Eastern Iowa horse rescue. I had called the rescue's go-to woman Kathy (not her real name), who recruited a parade of trucks with horse trailers for the day, as we were told there would be almost two dozen horses and nothing else. Danny drove the truck and trailer. Ask no more of him. Smart man. Danny and I were chatting, trying to make the two-hour ride go quickly. He kept checking his mirrors, and I kept turning my head to see through the back window into the bed of the truck, looking for evidence that anyone had awakened. I was feeling okay about how it was going so I decided to catch up with some phone calls I needed to make. When......

Just after getting off a four-lane highway, Danny and I both saw the male cougar's head pop up out of his crate.   (The crate was closest to the cab of the truck and up against the front side of the truck bed.) His face was pressed up against the glass of the back window and he was pushing upwards, trying to get himself out from the crate, but it was too close to the cab of the truck. I remember saying, "Oh shit, shit, shit, SHIT!" to the person I was speaking to on the phone, and throwing the phone down. While the truck slowed to a stop, I threw open the truck door, then jumped into the back to sit on the bouncing crate. By now the cougar was really frustrated and showing me every one of his beautiful canine teeth. With me on top of the crate, and the little sedation still left in him, he was not able to get out. His head was held in place between the crate and cab. I had so many things going through my mind, including, "How did I get to this point?!" along with headlines reading, "**Neglected Cougar Escapes Botched Rescue**."

Maybe you all want to know a bit more about the situation, like where did these animals even come from? I'll back track for you:

Several counties away, a rural Iowa couple kept four cougars, a black bear, and multiple horses, dogs, and cats. For a three year period the local shelter had been attempting to confiscate the animals after many reports of poor care. There were some cats in a little out-building living in heavily soiled floors, themselves soiled. There were 4 totally declawed cougars (also called mountain lions) in concrete pens, 24 intact dogs who were skin and bones, 11 emaciated horses, a fox, and chickens. And there was an adult black bear who had lived 6 years in a 10 by 10 foot chain-link dog pen, the last 3 of those years without having his pen cleaned, since his owners had boarded up the cage door (they were tired of him getting out). His only "toy" was a portion of a big metal barrel he had to turn over himself so the owners could put water in it for him to drink.

You may be thinking to yourself "WTF!?" Bear with me. (Ha! Pun!) This was rural Iowa. Up until 2008 **anyone** could purchase **any kind** of animal and keep it legally in the state of Iowa. To prove how stupid this was I will tell you where the bear came from. The owners' 18 year old son bought him at an auction 6 years previously when he was a cub. B-Bear was also 4-paw declawed and was a fun little pet the first few months. Once he got bigger they put him into the dog pen. Three years later the son died of a meth overdose. The parents had trouble containing B-Bear, who would get the gate off the pen and escape. Their solution was to literally board over the gate opening and nail it shut. How well was the door boarded? It took two large men using hammers and crowbars a good half hour to move it far enough for us to all carry the bear out. Three years of feces at the base was a big part of why the bottom was stuck.

So, as you'll recall, I was not experienced with this kind of stuff. But when a rescue group has the assistance of the local police in removing animals, state law requires a vet to be present. It's no different than getting all the planets aligned -- doesn't happen often. So as the only vet willing to help, I was the "it girl". I drew up a dosage of sedatives I had researched the night before and while the owners of B-Bear were getting "kisses" from him, (That is why they claimed he "loved" them! They pressed their faces to the chain-link and let him lick them. Damn bear was bored out of his skull! Of course he'll lick anything you put near him!) I slowly walked in, poked B-Bear in the butt, and backed up quickly.

I was out of the pen and the large men held the bulk of the "door" against the gate opening while we watched him go down. I held my breath. Last thing I wanted to do was kill a bear that had just spent the last three 3 living on his own shit. I wanted to do well by him.

All you experienced zoo vets, I would have handed this over to you in a second. Remember, the county had been trying for years to get these animals off the property. When asked to help, I assumed that first, they had already asked experienced vets. Maybe they did but couldn't afford one? Second, I assumed they had transportation for the animals. And third, I thought they had a place for the animals to go. They had none of those things. I vowed that next time I'm asked to help with exotic animals I will ask simple things like, "Will I be present solely for my veterinary skills? Do you just need my sign-off on their being removed? Or will I be in charge of relocating and housing the most difficult animals?"

Thankfully B-Bear went down smoothly. Once sleeping I examined him quickly to be sure he had a strong pulse and was breathing. When I was sure he was alive, yet asleep, I did a cursory physical exam. The most startling thing about B-Bear was his sad paws. Though they were stunningly big, I was saddened by the lack of claws and noted how soft and almost swollen the pads of his feet were due to his "bedding" of the last 3 years. We then promptly moved B-Bear, via a huge tarp, into the horse trailer (brand new, by the way)   that Danny's pickup was towing.

While he was taken away I used my three-foot-long syringe pole to sedate the cougars which were each placed into large dog crates which were provided by the shelter, and which as you know were missing bolts!

Now we fast-forward to that pivotal moment in my life when I was face to face with the fact that I was part of a group that took animals from a poor situation and put them into another totally bad situation.

Sitting on top of the crate containing that very unhappy cougar, somehow I remembered that I still had syringes, hypodermic needles, and sedatives in my pocket, and grabbed the first thing I touched. Armed with a 23- gauge needle, I poked his nose a few times so he would pull his head back in. Once his head was in, I continued to sit on the cage with my foot wedged between the crate front and the wall of the truck bed. I drew up more of the drugs, hands shaking, let him push the crate door open again then waited for his big face, sharp teeth and all, to pop out. When it did, I gave the injection in his masseter (cheek) muscle.

Simultaneous to this, Danny very calmly asked, "Should I call 911?" I told him yes, and that a taser would be nice. By the time the deputy showed up, the cat was going down. He later explained he didn't have a taser, and that he could shoot the cat if it escaped. I then pictured the headlines again — **"Really Screwed Up 'Rescue' Does More Harm than Good."**

That may seem like the end of the craziness. Nope. Remember I said three week period. Go ahead and go back to the first paragraph of this chapter and check to see if I'm lying. It will make the story seem longer too

Once back on the road, Danny continued driving in his casual way, as though he had not just witnessed an absolutely crazy escape attempt. I got back on the phone and began begging people to help take in the four cougars and bear temporarily. They were still legally owned by the people who wanted to go to court to fight for them, so were not in need of permanent homes yet. My first call was to the director of a local municipal shelter. "Pleeeaaaase. Could you take the cougars in for the next 24 hours?" I begged and pleaded. She agreed to 24 hours. They ended up staying over a week before being transferred to a rescue in Minnesota, for a while. (Ooh, foreshadowing.)

B-Bear was sitting pretty in the multi-horse trailer, so had no problems spending the night in it, parked in a barn at our best friends' farm a few miles away. After the near escape of the cougar we were terrified B-Bear would somehow get out of the trailer, then the barn and start wandering around Johnson County. We were so relieved the next morning to see his big dumb head partially sticking out of the trailer window.....which used to have bars on it....and glass. Yes, the first night the bear tore the bars off the trailer windows after first breaking the glass. He also managed to bend some bars on dividers that were meant to help separate the horses in the trailer. They were swung back along the wall pre-B-Bear, and were no longer post-B-Bear.

As mentioned earlier, the trailer was brand new. It had also been borrowed from someone who expected it would be used for, say, horses. Kathy had saved the day for us by getting it for us, but got in trouble after B-Bear's assault.

Eventually, on day 3, B-Bear was transported to a sanctuary in Davenport where he would proceed to bend and break and disfigure the cage he was in until it was almost useless. The facility called and said B-Bear had done so much destruction to a cage that had previously only housed big cats that she feared he would escape. B-Bear was coming back.

I was in panic mode. I had less than 24 hours to find a place for a 400 lb. bear who liked to bend metal. (In case you are wondering how a simple dog pen held him all those years, I have to tell you he did indeed chew his way out once. The original cage was subsequently covered with the heaviest gauge chain-link available, making it a double-walled pen, except of course at the spot with the huge hole he chewed out of it.) At the time I was officially working in my mobile vet practice, Animals All About Inc., but was pulling Witty Kitties, our special-needs shelter, into the fray. Witty Kitties was becoming better known and we had a handful of volunteers who lived close and were amazingly loyal. We had just moved Witty Kitties' cats out of our garage and into their new and current location in a huge metal building on our property. Torben and I actually had the garage back. But did we need it, really?

Yep, I decided to put B-Bear in our two-car garage. To hell with protecting our cars.

I immediately called Torben, our best friends, and Witty Kitties volunteers, asking if everyone could come help gut the garage. I had to work the following day. I had to say no more. That day, between surgeries, I made phone calls to find out what type of metal gate or fencing could be used to put over the windows and along the walls of the garage. The garage was single-walled (no insulation or interior wall) so seemed like something B-Bear could chew through easily if bored. I found that the 14 foot long panels used in bull pens would do. I ordered them. With the help of a guy who used to work at the municipal shelter, I arranged for a rental truck so they could be picked up at the local farm supply store. At the same time an army of volunteers, many I had never met before showed up at my house. With the direction of our best friends, they removed every item from the garage, took down all the shelves, and removed the glass from the windows.

By the time I got home it was completely cleared. This was a moment that really touched me because I bet everyone there may have had more fun things to do than clean out a garage. It didn't occur to me they may have been excited about the possibility of seeing a huge bear.

First thing the next morning I remember calling a big supporter of ours. She had recently donated a large amount to Witty Kitties. I don't remember WHY I called her, but was talking a mile-a-minute about the past few days and how I was headed down to Iowa City to pick up panels to line our garage, and oh my God I was going on and on and on. "Jenni," she said calmly. I babbled on while taking the exit off I80 into Iowa City. "Jenni. I will send you a check for...." I was like "What?" "I will send you a check for..." I was stunned and gushing with gratitude. You see, heavy bull panels are not cheap. Repairs for a horse trailer are not cheap. I even felt I needed to send money to the Davenport woman for damages. I will be eternally grateful to Jane for that. She is still a constant at most of the functions in the area where any sort of animal cause is involved.

So B-Bear arrived that night. We were all super nervous as he walked slowly down the ramp from the smaller horse trailer provided by the woman. (Why can't I remember her name?) We had all the volunteers, most of them young twenty-somethings, holding wooden panels up to provide him an aisle through which to walk. No one knew how he would behave and imagined him going off on a rampage and knocking someone over. Nope, he sauntered in, we shut the garage door, and he was at his new temporary home.

Having B-Bear was extremely rewarding to us. He had never had so much space. He had never been in a bathtub in his adult life either. When he got into it and sat and splashed over and over again I felt like crying.

Over the next few weeks we learned he could turn a car tire inside out. He could knock Torben down with a slight push of the forepaw even though Torben is 6' 2" and was 220 lbs. And, he could very easily bend that damned bull paneling, without claws! A friend, Virginia, who was in her early 70's at the time, came with a gift for Ben. She brought him a rubber ball, the type you see in the huge baskets at the toy store, or at the end of the aisle at Target. She tossed it to B-Bear, then "pop!" the moment B-Bear grabbed it with his mouth. "Well, that was fun," said Virginia in her no nonsense, matter-of-fact way.

A less funny feat by B-Bear was tearing out the capped end of the propane pipe that had fed the heater back when the building was our Witty Kitties shelter. The outrageous odor seeping out of the garage greeted me when I got home that evening. I was thankful no one in our family smokes, that the windows of the garage had no glass, and that the naughty B-Bear was alive and conscious.

Jenni, this still sounds like just a fun story. At the beginning of the chapter you promised, or at least mentioned, this was a really crazy stupid story. OK, here you go.

The county had a huge legal case against the cougar/B-Bear people: photos, videos, reports from five other veterinarians who looked at the malnourished dogs and cats from the property. I had my reports in order. The sheriff and two deputies all had reports confirming the horrible conditions of the property and animals. The local humane society, which took responsibility for housing the dogs and cats thank God, had reports. Kathy and I arrived at the courthouse all ready and raring to go. (Kathy came mostly as a hugely good friend.) Sitting in the county attorney's office, all the supporting cast members were talking about how much of a no-brainer the case would be. We were ready to testify.

The county attorney talked to us. He barely glanced at the pictures and reports and asked how sure we were the people should be charged with neglect. We confirmed our positions. He abruptly left the room for a few minutes.........then came back. "They're all going back...except the bear, chickens, and fox. They don't want those." It was over.

We all looked at each other. WTF? Did we hear that right? "Wait, what?" I asked. "The animals are all going back." For reasons even he wouldn't give the county attorney, whom I will call Dick, gave all the animals the couple wanted back to them without setting eyes on a single photo or the video from the raid. The judge wasn't even willing to examine the case or look at pictures because there would be no case! He simply did what Dick recommended and signed the papers saying the people would not be charged with cruelty or neglect. This meant the county was now going to have to return all the animals except the "throwaways" the people no longer wanted (how convenient!) — the bear, chickens, and fox.

There was absolutely **nothing** we could do. Could we talk to the judge? No. Not allowed. I called all the bigger Iowa organizations asking what we could do. The attorney was evil as far as I was concerned. The law enforcement and other animal welfare folks were

49

equally dismayed. I did eventually get the story from one of the deputies as to why Dick was being such a DICK. Dick had just lost a re-election bid. He was out. What did he care about the animals and the huge bill the county was now going to have to pay for all the housing and veterinary services for all these animals. We are talking many of thousands of dollars.

Kathy and I drove home together absolutely livid. I raged and yelled. I had to keep from speeding, my adrenalin was so high. At one point my cell phone rang. Back then I still talked on the phone when on fast roads. I saw it was Torben. Good. I get to vent to someone new. I hit the "talk" button and without saying "hi" I just went into "Oh my GOD. You would not fucking believe what happened! They got the animals back. The Attorney is a baby who just wanted to.....,"

Then I heard "Jenni! JENNI! B-Bear is.....(Indecipherable).....!"

"What? What?"

"B-Bear----is----getting---**out**!" He was obviously struggling. "Call.....! Call ....!"

Not known to me, at the other end of the phone "line" Torben was standing on the outside of our garage struggling hard to push B-Bear back in. Torben had been mowing the lawn when he noticed B-Bear's head and a paw waving about through the window. Torben, being Torben, never puts contacts into his phone, so could call the only number he knew, me. I then quickly called two of our closest neighbors. They came to the rescue. One said later that he had just driven past moments before and saw Torben at the window seeming to "play" with B-Bear and thought nothing of it. With aid, Torben was able to contain B-Bear again.

So, at the end of the day we owned a bear, and were owed thousands of dollars by the county. The same county also owed all the other animal organizations for the care (husbandry and medical) of all the other animals as well. The county attorney had left them with a bill "F.U." of a bill. It was a battle for all of us to collect even a fraction of the total cost. Fortunately, generous donations offset our expenses and allowed us to donated to the groups who had temporarily housed the cougars and B-Bear.

I am happy to say two years later, Kathy, I, and our most loyal Witty Kitties volunteers, ran around the Iowa State Capital building lobbying folks to vote for a new exotic animal restriction law. I truly believe my showing the picture of B-Bear to senators and representatives and saying "This bear was purchased and owned legally by an 18 year old boy...." That caught their attention.

Fortunately the law passed, and now a special permit is required to own bears, tigers, lions, etc. Of course, as is typical with the government, plans for how to enforce the new law were not in place and many people still have them. But it's a start.

Today B-Bear lives at an incredible sanctuary in Florida with two female bears. Almost 3 months after he arrived at our home, the sanctuary staff arrived in a large truck that towed an enormous air conditioned trailer behind it. They very professionally lured him into a sturdy custom-made metal cage which was then rolled up a ramp into his ride home. Raw whole chicken (the ones our dog Buster did not steal while we weren't watching) and marshmallows were all they needed to make him do what they wanted. Once at his new home, he had to be neutered before introduction to his new gals; but besides that, I think he must be the happiest a Bear can be considering his beginnings.

Almost two years after B-Bear arrived at his new home, Torben, Kirsten and I visited the sanctuary. B-Bear was a great distance from us, foraging in his environment. I called him, and couldn't believe he came running! I was so happy. But several yards away from us he stopped, did a little hoppy dance, and started eating something off the ground. "I threw blueberries over there." His caretaker said. That was it. B-Bear had berries, girlfriends, and space, and forgot about me. I was grateful for that.

The Best of Times. The Worst of Times

As I was spaying yet another animal, the billionth of the day, I tried to gather my thoughts once more. I was at a humane society I serviced every other week, and trying to enjoy the peace and quiet in the small clinic behind the shelter building, while deciding what drugs to use on the next dog that needed my attention. I was having a little trouble on this day, however. After just a bit of thinking as to why, I looked down at the two tiny arms wrapped around my legs that were attached to a tiny person who was screaming and crying, "Momma. Mommmmmm-mmmaa. Momma!" It was uncanny how Kirsten could detect just when I was least available, and decide that was the best time to need me desperately. Hadn't I just taken her out in her stroller? Luckily the six rocks I found in a pile by the driveway preoccupied her for a good half hour. After those got boring, stacking eight cans of dog food kept her happy, until that moment. Her behavior wasn't unusual since she was only almost 2 years old.

I have to confess I behaved in a similar way with my own mom back when I was maybe 2….or 12 years old. My mom had seven of us by the age of 30, so had numerous hands clinging to her much of her life. I remember the highlight of her day had dwindled down to stealing away to the only bathroom in the house armed with a cup of coffee, her cigarettes, and a crossword puzzle. She would stay in there for the better part of an hour. That doesn't mean we didn't try to ruin her bit of solitude by standing directly outside the bathroom door, whining the whole time. The piano was right there. I'd park my butt on the piano stool and complain, "Mom. Mommmmmmm. Mom!" Sound familiar? Maybe she had earplugs hidden away in there too. The gall of taking time away from us was too much to bear. How selfish.

But I'll get back to the inappropriate use of surgical space as a childcare facility. I was not alone in my crazy dilemma of having to work on animals at the same time as care for a kid. I have known plenty of mom veterinarians in the same situation. Many times I've put my little tyke into a large dog kennel (a clean one!) to provide her with a safe play area while I was working on tricky animals. People who've witnessed this may have thought of calling DHS, but I defy anyone to find a safer playpen than a 3 x 3 x 3 foot stainless steel cage, stuffed full of blankets and toys. This care technique has been used numerous times by moms who needed just a bit of time to do their work unencumbered, quickly and methodically working through the situation. It is an act of necessity.

I felt my blood pressure rise as I tried to concentrate on the task at hand (surgery!) while still reserving a small part of my brain to direct my mouth to sing "The Wheels on the Bus" at the top of my lungs just one more time. I wondered how I got to this point in my life. But I never wonder over the question for long, as I know very well that my life is just as I've made it to be . . . and want it to be . . . as full of life as possible. I can look back at so many situations in my past, both extremely happy and devastatingly sad, thanks to my strong desire to take care of animals, especially the rejected misfits, and realize that I wouldn't change a thing. Although getting our baby into daycare will be a blessing, these situations are an integral part of my family's days. However, anyone seeing them from the outside may just want to run and get a movie camera, as they could easily win a prize on "America's Funniest Videos!"

For instance, there was the time when I had to use a plumbing snake to unplug our toilet. I wasn't the least bit surprised when I saw pieces of starfish, shells and sand dollars coming out. I had discovered not long before that one of the raccoons we had been rehabilitating had learned how to flush the toilet and had been playing in it. I just wish I had had the sense to remove the glass bowl of sea creatures from the back of the tank. That raccoon (the thought of her still makes my heart swell), Junie B. Coonie, was the source of innumerable fun moments and some frustrations. She was from one of a few batches of baby coons we had taken in due to separation from their mothers for various reasons. Though we released them into the wild on our 14 acres, Junie knew very well that boxes of cereal, bags of white rice, and rolls of toilet paper were waiting for her in our house. They were just begging to be opened, dragged around the house, and played with! The wild of the forest was nice, but after about a week out there she insisted on coming in through the dog/cat door and welcoming herself back into our lives.

Junie especially liked to hit the bedrooms first, at night of course, and to try to reach her fingers as far into our ears or nostrils as possible. Our hair was always in need of being messed up, and she also insisted on one or two of our dogs joining in the fun. I may be the only mom in Iowa who heard her son yelling, "Mom, the raccoon keeps bugging me" in the middle of the night. We all had different tolerances for Junie. Though she was the most personable, sweet, cuddly little muffin you could ever meet, she was still a wild animal, so she had an "anything goes" attitude in our house. Torben was certainly the most tolerant. But Joseph (my son) and I got especially frustrated with her night raids.

We really got fed up when she entered our house after a long while away in late December to discover we had brought in a tree just for her, and decorated it with shiny lights and play things all over. We had even put fun boxes covered with colorful paper that ripped easily, and ribbons that made the boxes easy to drag away. We really had the nerve to think it was our Christmas tree, and shouldn't have been surprised when dozens of decorations started disappearing at a fast rate. We also had to stop putting presents under the tree. Junie, despite her opposable thumbs, couldn't shake the presents to find out what was inside, so had to tear them apart. To this day, I think she taught our terrier Cha Cha her quick "retrieval and entry" technique for opening any kind of package.

Needless to say, I was thrilled when I figured out how to scare Junie from the tree. (Spray her with water? Are you joking? Yell at her to scare her? You're ridiculous!) I had plugged a vacuum cleaner into a nearby outlet and left the vacuum in the "on" position. I put an adapter at the plug site to control the vacuum's switch with a remote control, allowing me to actually turn it on and off from another room. Thus I appeared completely innocent and sympathetic, of course, when she sprang 3 feet in the air and hightailed it back out to the woods when the evil vacuum erupted into a deafening noise. I admit, I've always had a bit of regret and sadness when seeing this in my mind, as I loved Junie so much, and I hated thinking she may one day never visit again. Even though Junie's leaving forever was supposed to be the ultimate outcome to our having raised her, I would have a mix of happiness and anger when I'd come home and discover she had come back. I would know she had been in the house because I would find everything previously on the kitchen table now on the floor.

Junie isn't the only raccoon who entertained us as well as caused hours of frustration. When Junie and her three buddies were still feeding off baby bottles, Torben and I took them on a camping trip to southern Illinois. A few hours into the adventure we decided to let them run loose in the van, as they were getting the crate all poopy and smelly. As long as we made sure none were near the driver's pedals, everything would be okay, right? Well, about an hour after a pit stop we noticed none of the coonies were visible. To make matters worse, a small sliding window in the back of the van was partially open. We immediately began taking the van apart. One, two, three, but where is the fourth? A good 30 minutes into the search, I found him inside the back seat, sleepy and annoyed for being bothered. Back into the crate they went. I have wonderful photos of that trip, the four of them playing at an overlook at a nature preserve, climbing the benches and scaring each other. The weathered wood, contrasting with their beautiful coats, made for some great shots. Of course, I also remember with joy the pictures I have of them when they spent the night loose in our bathroom. All the drawers and cupboards were open and the trash was tipped over. Towels and toilet paper were strewn all over the place. Their first experience "hunting" for live crayfish in a kiddie pool was probably the pinnacle of cute. Oh yeh, did I mention how they crawled up our bare legs first thing each morning while waiting for their bottles?

My point is that my life is a mess! I have no personal time to think of anything, I am always doing ten projects at a time, and I lie awake at night worrying about what I've forgotten to do. Why, it was only last week when I was stopped at a light in Coralville by a cab driver, only to be told I had a stack of towels and a box on the bumper of my 24 ft. veterinary van. The fact that they were there isn't so weird -- for me, that is. The crazy thing is that they survived the 15 mile trip from my home! Just another day. . . I complain with the best of them, but when I try to picture my life any other way, I can't. I love how things are, and I don't have many regrets. I just need a bit of fine-tuning . . . okay, a lot of fine-tuning!

Does Nature Take Its Course Anymore?

I went to sleep last night thinking about a Canada goose I had put down earlier in the evening. It was really sad, but waiting wasn't going to help her. The longer I waited, the longer she suffered. She was taken from the Iowa River in Iowa City a few days ago, after being chipped away from the ice she was frozen to. Two days before, another goose had been taken away the same way. That one hadn't survived the rescue.

After taking her home, I got to wondering if this was the mate of the first goose. If so, will it eat? Was it sick already, and therefore unable to swim about and keep from getting frozen into the ice? I slowly warmed her and waited till the next day to really check her out. It was pretty apparent she had neurological issues. Starvation? Liver? Lead? Trauma? In just two days she went from being able to stand, to only being able to sit up, to then being unable to hold her head in a normal position. When it comes to wildlife, I am not big on working up possible medical issues as most of them are in the process of dying and humans just happen to find them while on their way out. They usually are hard cases to solve as standard lab blood values haven't been established in most species. Mind you, in trauma cases it is different: Animal is hurt. Find out how. Can you fix it? Fix it if you can. Fairly straightforward.

But I digress.

I woke up in the middle of the night wondering about the goose, only to doze off, until awakened in the morning by my clock radio. The story I woke to was Iowa Public Radio's coverage of another pair of geese being chipped from the same river.

So now I'm thinking that the Department of Natural Resources needs to get involved at this point. Is there something "going around?" Maybe this is natural old age in a flock. But I got to thinking; the fact that they're sitting in a river in a large city likely meant something environmental was going on, possibly the fault of humans. If so, did that make it natural?

What does that mean? "Natural."

The first time I ever thought phrases like "Let's just let nature take its course," or, "I like my animals to be the way nature meant them to be" were stupid was during my first year as a veterinarian.

After vet school, I got a job at a clinic in a somewhat rural bedroom community of western Washington State. I was getting acquainted with the clientele, and learning that the spectrum of people ranged from, "Gee, I'd rather put a bullet in that cat's head before putting $25 into it," to, "Do absolutely everything you can. Money isn't an object." The latter was true only half the time. For the other half, indeed money was an object. Unfortunately, it was often hard to tell which group we were dealing with until after handing over the bill and finding the owners hadn't a cent. I got chewed out by my boss a lot for falling for clients' earnest pleas to do anything at any cost, only to find they couldn't afford what they'd agreed to have done.

There was a guy in his thirties that taught me that nature really has little to do with anything. He was arguing with me because I was STRONGLY urging him to let me spay his very pregnant golden retriever. Let me tell you why. This dog had become pregnant the previous summer also, by her older half-brother. Both of them suffered from idiopathic epileptic seizures and had passed it on to their babies. The owner had trouble finding them homes, and hadn't even considered having the pups neutered, either. I expressed how difficult it would be finding homes for yet more epileptic dogs, not to mention how stressful this all was for the pregnant dog, who was not yet two years old. He reasoned that since the puppies usually didn't show signs of seizures till a few years of age, he would give them away, letting the new owners discover whether they would eventually have seizures. Nice. His other reasoning was, "You just want my money. I don't think it is natural to take away their parts."

I had to hold my breath and think before finally saying, "OK, number one... Golden retrievers aren't 'natural.' They are the result of specific breeding over many, many years by people who decided to do so based on whatever arbitrary trait they liked about them. Along with the wonderful traits came bad ones, like hereditary epilepsy. They are domesticated. They are people's product, not nature's."

He looked at me like I was an over-educated idiot who was trying to do her evil deeds to his beloved dog. He left the office without anything being resolved.

The good news is he did schedule the spay after talking to my boss, who fortunately told him I wasn't an idiot. But the bad news is that he waited another two weeks into the pregnancy. The poor dog was ready to burst. But, believing in my heart it was best, I did spay the then very near-term pregnant dog, thus terminating the lives of 13 babies. It was miserable, messy, sad, and horrible. I kept wondering which of them would have been OK and not been epileptic, and which wouldn't.

I can assure those people still bearing with me and reading this that there was no suffering for the puppies. The anesthetic drugs used on the mother dog affect the babies as well. They remain in the uterus and do not feel cold or the pain of a needle. Their blood supply is simply cut off. Because they do not breathe oxygen (no functioning lungs yet), they don't "gasp for air." It is an entirely sad thing to do but I kept in mind the sadness for dogs that experience frequent seizure episodes. At the time phenobarbital with potassium bromide was the treatment of choice for epileptic animals. The potential damage to the liver from chronic phenobarbital required monitoring drug blood levels and liver function. At that time I didn't know a soul who would have taken on a dog like that. Now, 25 years later, I know quite a few, but that is hindsight.

This case was especially hard because golden retrievers are my all-time favorite breed. My first and favorite and most loyal dog ever was a golden. I hope to have another someday should a needy one cross my path when I'm not already in possession of four dogs. But if some of you still think I'm callous, I must tell you it is heart-breaking to euthanize a happy dog who doesn't understand that his owner needs to do so because the expense of treating the seizures, doing routine blood work, and still witnessing frequent seizures has become too unbearable for the family.

A year had not gone by since meeting the man with the golden retrievers before the "nature" issue arose again. It was this event that almost kept me from helping an animal rescue group again.

I alluded to this story in the first chapter. I had taken in one of the few truly feral cats I've ever dealt with from a local group I'll not name. It was a terrified little female tabby not even a year old. She had been in a trap for three days before being brought in to the clinic as no one was able to deal with her. She was my first jab-while-still-in-the-trap cat. Once anesthetized, I examined and radiographed her. She had a fractured pelvis with soft tissue damage to the spinal cord. Because of this, she could not pee on her own. Her bladder would be in a constant state of being full. Once pressure built up to a critical point, a little urine would come out, but she could never empty her bladder beyond about 80%. Long story short, if left, the kidneys would eventually fail. Oh, and until then, she would be in a lot of pain.

Thus began the daily manual expressing of her bladder, something that should have been done several times a day. But because she was so wild, she had to be sedated heavily each time, so it could reasonably be done only once or twice daily. This was no easy task. Each time I approached her cage, she climbed to the top and hung there, using her forelegs, mostly due to the weakened state of her back end. She'd thrash and strike and growl. All the while I knew she had to be absolutely terrified of me. So, I'd sedate her with the syringe at the end of the stick or else net her and roll her up. It took only twice to convince me her pelvis was never going to heal this way. I mentioned as much to the "rescue" group, but was met with, "Well then we'll take her home."

Worried that the group would not express her bladder, I kept her in the clinic another three days. I hoped she would miraculously gain the ability to urinate on her own. That didn't happen. Each time I emptied it the bladder was a huge tight ball, and I needed to put a lot of pressure on it before any urine came out. She ate not a bit. I doubt she drank either. It was hard to tell because she trashed her cage constantly. I had to give her subcutaneous fluids while she was sedated to prevent dehydration, which wasn't helping her kidneys. The almost constant pressure from the excess urine in the bladder put pressure on the kidneys, which could damage them. Also the residual urine in the bladder (I could never get it totally emptied) could allow stagnation and bacterial growth. These could lead to kidney failure, toxicity, and then death.

I finally expressed my concern for the cat's physical state, as well as her psyche, to the "rescue" group. I tried to make them understand that the cat was a young, terrified little thing who only knew fear and pain at the moment. Treatment and human handling only made it worse. I suggested euthanizing her.

I wasn't prepared for the barrage of words that followed. I was cruel, unfeeling, inhumane, and unfit to care for any of their animals ever again (that last one I agreed with). The mere suggestion of euthanasia, which by definition is a humane death free of pain and fear, went against everything they believed in. They took the cat back, saying they would "let nature take its course." From what I heard it did. It took a few days before the poor thing died. Whether from lack of food, water, or failure of her kidneys, I don't know. I CAN say the cat surely suffered. The "rescue" did not allow for a humane death.

That was the first of two times I decided animal rescue people were too crazy to work with, and swore them off forever. Of course, it didn't work either time.

A more recent dilemma was when I agreed to take in two young female coyotes many Julys ago. They had been orphaned shortly after birth and raised for six weeks in a home where they lived as "house dogs," and played with the family's cocker spaniel. Assuming a rehabilitator would have no problem getting them into the wild again, Torben and I took them in without a second thought. Unfortunately, we had them another two weeks before finding a rehabber who could give us advice, though wasn't able to take them. We learned it was possible to teach them the ways of the wild and provide a "soft release" into the wild; but our heavily wooded 14 acres is surrounded by neighbors, some who thought we were awesome and others who thought we were hoarders who went out of our way to collect animals. A few zoo-type places were willing to take them, but their enclosures were not much more than dog runs. We couldn't take them across state lines legally and I was worried about doing anything that would tarnish our reputation (not that we never did, but more about that later).

Scoopy and Minnie (as we named them) were too young in my opinion to be released after their domestic puppyhood. Yet it would be winter by the time they came of age and could be let into the wild. In the meantime, the question was, would we be able to give them an environment that restricted our contact and kept them from associating us with food? While pondering this I just started building a cage. In a matter of days, they were finally running around in an approximately 40 x 60 foot pen with 6 foot high fencing and an additional foot, curved inward at the top, that would inhibit climbing out. I also put fencing flat on the ground and attached it to the bottom of the fence to prevent digging. The highlight of the pen was that we built it around a two-story tree house with stairs that they could enjoy climbing.

During morning chores, it was wonderful seeing the coyotes atop the tree house platforms, watching the geese and ducks, hoping another one of the birds would accidently fly into their pen. They ran and scampered and fought and played to their hearts' content. Environment enrichment could be fun for me as well. I loved taping up boxes with treats inside for them to tear apart. We gave them a great variety of toys and foods. Some mornings when they weren't interested in coming near me, I'd just lie on the ground and let them circle me until they were brave enough to take their food from my hand. In the evenings, they seemed more than happy to jump on my back and grab my hair or clothes.

It soon became obvious to us all that the coyotes were with us to stay. Once that decision was made, we learned the more we were able to interact with them, the better. So that is what we did.

But it wasn't a painless decision. Were we depriving them of a life they would have preferred? I have heard many opinions telling me it was cruel to keep them and that I should have tried to put them out into the wild so they could do what was natural. Natural? Their mother was killed accidently by a human. Natural? No. If I let them go after already having become comfortable as pups with the human world, would they get hit by a car? Shot? Starve? I got to thinking about where on this planet I could let them run wild without humans being an issue. When a coyote is hit on the road, it isn't natural as far as I'm concerned. And it's not painless by any means. So why would I let them go out and risk that? How many acres would it take? One of the best rehabilitators in the area is only 2 miles from the city. She has a wonderful acreage, but she admits the proximity can be a problem.

I had to release other wildlife we had rehabilitated in the past. It is always hard because they go out into the dangerous unknown. Most of the baby squirrels or possums or raccoons we've taken in were orphaned due to a mom being hit by a car, shot by a gun, killed by a pet dog, or killed by a tree being felled by a chainsaw. How natural is that? I wonder just how much of this natural business is really going on. Deer are hit on roads. Do we shoot them to lessen this, hopefully preventing the suffering of those that don't die immediately? Do we let them starve due to overpopulation? Or do we shoot them to lessen their numbers? Where IS this line of natural vs. unnatural?

I don't believe we were wrong for keeping the coyotes, but we were not right either. The decision was based on the situation, simply the one we made at the time. Having made that decision, we worked hard to give Scoopie and Minnie as interesting a life as we could with as much room to roam as possible. I was torn knowing how much ground coyotes in the wild can cover in a day. Ours did get plenty of hunting practice thanks to the periodic animals that made their way into the pen. I found numerous dead squirrels, and even mice, lying on the ground. Not sure if the coyotes eventually ate them, but I often caught them playing catch with them on their own.

What I have learned is that there is no such thing as natural where humans live so close to wild areas. We humans interact and affect wildlife whether we want to or not. Our decisions to intervene with injured or orphaned feral animals could be called interfering with nature. Or it could be just our attempt to undo the unnatural damage we have done that causes such things to happen. No one can tell me convincingly they know all the answers to that one.

Anyway, so here I am, almost 25 years after my first interaction with that crazy rescue group, the one that convinced me those "do-gooder-animal-folks" are insane. I still feel there is a small percentage of them that will never understand that sometimes we intervene to save, and sometimes to kill humanely when the only other option is continued suffering. Sometimes we set the nursed-to-health animal free again, and sometimes we keep them for life.

Obviously I've changed my mind about dealing with rescue groups as I've found people doing rescues come in all forms. My first shelter experience in Iowa ended up being a major disaster because the woman in charge was extremely self-serving and dysfunctional. On the other hand, a shelter in Utah and subsequent rescues and shelters in Iowa have involved, for the most part, wonderful people who all just want to do what is right for the animals, egos aside. So, of course I changed my mind and now work right along as one of them. Yeah, I changed my mind.

Naturally.

No Flowers for Mother's Day

On Mother's Day in 2011, I broke a big promise I made to Joseph a few years earlier. It involved something I was getting for Mother's Day. You would think a son would be happy if his mom already knew what she wanted, so he wouldn't have to wonder what to get for her. Sons want to please moms, right? I did not insist on flowers or candy or brunch from him, but I knew he still wanted me to have a nice day. So he should have been happy for me and the gift I was about to receive, at no monetary cost to him. I'm a simple girl. I was getting a 400 pound black bear.

Joseph has a memory a billion times more accurate than mine, and when I told him we were taking in a second bear he fumed and said, "Mom! You specifically (he very carefully enunciated each syllable so my daft brain understood) said after B-Bear left that you would get no more bears!" With complete honesty I calmly replied, "No I didn't. Why would I say something like that?" I said it with complete honesty because I had absolutely no memory of saying it. However, as we conversed back and forth, son as parent, parent as child, I began to recall making the promise. I can almost remember thinking, what were the chances of my ever coming across another bear that needed a home come my way?

Poor Joseph. I knew he was right, even though I didn't remember saying such a thing. I am sure I did, and meant it. But I just didn't remember. After more arguing, I told him we had a place for the bear already, the approximately 50 by 60 foot pen Joseph and I had built to keep the two young coyotes in. The fencing was pretty heavy, but I knew it needed reinforcing and planned to add 6 foot tall chain link panels to the outside of the fence. Joseph was disgusted with me. I told him all I wanted from him as a gift was to stay silent and non-critical about my present-to-come. Knowing he wouldn't do a good job of this, he didn't take the day off from work on Mother's Day, which was okay. Who can blame him for his inability to keep his mouth shut when I add craziness to our lives? I accept the fact that my inundation with animals has put him off ever wanting any for himself.

Ben was a 20 year old black bear who lived with another bear in a circular corncrib at a petting zoo just east of the Quad Cities. The other black bear had died. The owners were getting older, and they no longer kept a license for the animals. We learned of Ben through a mutual friend who had known Ben since he was a cub, and even had the chance to feed him with a baby bottle when the people first acquired him. After much deliberation, we decided to take him on. We had really enjoyed having B-Bear for a short time six years earlier, and still thought of him a lot.

Once we agreed to take Ben, I began to worry. First, there was the promise I had made Joseph. I'm not sure whether he insisted on me making that promise because he was concerned about safety, or just didn't want people to think his mom was a freak. I was worried because he was really stressed out by the decision. Over dinner one evening I tried to calm him by telling him what animals we were *not* taking from the petting zoo: orangutan, capuchin monkey, baboons, and others. "Oh, God!" he responded. He probably now feared there was a chance I would be coming home with those too.

I have always taken in pretty much "anything," but primates are way too smart, dexterous, carry more zoonotic diseases than I am aware of, and so are just off limits. Also, we knew there was a chance Ben wouldn't be coming at all because the owners wanted to sell him. Torben and I were out of the animal buying stage in our life, so had refused to give them anything. We felt they should actually be the ones paying us, considering the money it would take to prepare for and keep him.

Finally, about the 1st of May, it was 99% a sure thing he was coming. So then the work started. Torben and I went to the farm supply store to order some big fence panels. Then I spent days reinforcing the coyote pen. We tried the panels on the inside of the pen first, but that didn't work out. Once I got them all up nicely on the outside, I had Torben come directly to the pen after work that day to do his "I'm-a-six-foot-tall-bear" act. He shook the walls. They were WAY too wobbly. So I bought long lag screws to attach boards on the outside for stability. After running out of boards and screws, I headed off to the lumber yard for more. This time I pulled in a volunteer, John, as he is cursed with owning an awesome pickup truck that has carried everything from alligators to bales of hay for these crazy people he has become involved with since his retirement. Putting the rest of the boards up made a world of difference. I was feeling pretty satisfied.

But that evening, Friday, two days before the bear was to arrive, I asked Torben to come down the hill after work to be my guinea pig-bear, putting the walls of the pen to the test by yanking and hanging on them. Torben was about 220 pounds, nowhere near the weight of an adult black bear, but the best I had to work with. Unfortunately (or fortunately) Torben had had a really bad week at work and was in as foul a mood as could be. So his act as pseudo-bear didn't take much effort. He went into the pen, shook the walls, then reached up to the fence overhanging the top of the pen and pulled it down, bending it and the rebar with little effort.

We both released a string of expletives before I ran off to the hardware store where I found only the same wimpy rebar. Larger diameter could be ordered, but who had the time to wait? I set out again for the farm supply store where I found 3/4 inch diameter rod. The problem was that they were much too long at 4 feet. Physics dictates a long bar is easier to bend than a short bar. How the heck was I going to cut 3/4 inch diameter metal rods? Then it dawned on me to call our neighbor Larry (as he shall be called). Larry is a great guy. We have absolutely nothing in common with regards to politics, religion, or various social issues. But he has always been great to talk to about that fact. And he is just a good man.

I called him from the store and said, "Larry, do you think you could cut some thick steel bars for me?" I was *certain* he would say he couldn't, once he heard how big they were. "Sure," he said easily. Relieved, I grabbed the rods, paid, and set out for Larry's house. He was outside with his grandkids and pretty much expecting me. When he saw the rods, he said, "What do you mean, can I cut those?" He laughed, got his band saw going, and quickly cut me multiple 2 foot sections of rod. After all the metal was cut, I went home and down the hill again. The pen finally got finished after working that evening and next morning on Saturday. Later that day, I talked to the folks with the bear who said it was a "go." "Damned right it is a go!" I thought to myself.

Once that was settled, the rock in my stomach sank, and my nerves started up again. I obsessed again about how we may be too naïve about our ability to keep a big old bear. Was I just romanticizing about how great it was to have B-Bear? Would the new bear try to kill the coyotes?

Mother's Day came. I got breakfast in bed from Kirsten, a protein bar and can of diet Pepsi. Say what you want. It really was what I wanted for breakfast. Kirsten gave me an acrylic painting that now hangs in our guest bathroom, and a pot in which she had planted sunflower seeds. Three had sprouted which pleased us both. That was pretty much it, except for Ben the Bear. Despite my happiness I had a nagging feeling in the back of my brain, and discovered Torben was having trouble relaxing as well. One thing we agreed on was that if we arrived at the place and decided to change our minds, we would just back out. Also, we needed a plan to get Ben through three gates, over our small water garden and down the hill.

This is where my friend, Kathy, entered the picture. Kathy already had experience with bears. It was she who kindly helped bring B-Bear to us. As usual, Kathy was willing to help again, taking a beautiful Sunday off to do so. Along for the ride was Danny, the very same guy I rode with the day the cougars almost got out of their crates while hauling them in the back of his pickup truck.

Though we had a history with Kathy and Danny, there they were again, ready to tackle another challenging animal. Kathy and Danny were in the front of the SUV and Torben, Kirsten, and I were in the back for the long drive to DeWitt. The questions and "devil's advocacy" from the front seat started as soon as we got out of our driveway. How would we do this? How would we do that? I actually appreciated it, if you can believe that, as I really didn't want to have anything go wrong just because we hadn't planned things beforehand.

We finally met Ben. He was in the back of his owner's horse trailer. He was breathing hard, making stressed sounds, and looking to get out. I didn't like any of that at all. But after being there a while, I noticed a small piece of hog paneling covering a large space at the top of the gate of the trailer. It was intact, not bent at all. Knowing B-Bear had been able to bend that stuff like a bendy-straw, I was happy to know that while sitting in the trailer for over 24 hours, Ben hadn't explored that big space to try to get out. It couldn't have been 5 feet high, a good sign.

We respected the fact that the owner, who had him since he was a cub, was cautious with him and never assumed Ben would be mellow 100% of the time. Once in a while he could get surly. When we were shown the little corncrib pen he had been in for all those years, I have to say I couldn't blame him. The structure was only 20 feet in diameter.

If this story were not so long, I'd tell you about the primates we saw. Alas, I'll stick with Ben's story. Besides, I'll be writing about us picking up the primates in a few years anyway. Kidding! Joseph wouldn't think that was a funny joke. But he doesn't read my stories anyway.

Finally we started the drive home. Again, brand-new questions kept coming from the front seat. There was second-guessing of every idea we had discussed before picking up Ben. I turned to Torben and mouthed the words, "I'm so nervous!" He mouthed back, "Me, too!" My stomach was a mess. I was wondering if this was a mistake. But towards the end of the long drive from DeWitt, Danny had a great idea for how to get Ben down the hill using the huge steel cage we bought from his former owners (they did get money from us after all). Danny wasn't planning to help, mind you. He was just the "idea man." We still had no idea how we would get the bear through the front yard with the little ponds. We entertained the idea of halting the mission and stopping at Danny's house where we could leave the bear while taking a few days to figure this problem out.

But again, I made a phone call, this time to John. He and our best friends were already heading to our house. I told him the plan we had and its glitches, then just hung up, hoping for them to do some magical thinking while we detoured to Danny's. Sure enough, after a surprisingly short amount of time, they figured out a solution to our biggest problem. So once we made it home it was time to move the big boy out.

This is what we did: Torben recruited two big guys from work, and with them we felt confident we had a good, strong group of people. Kathy backed the trailer as close to our front yard gate as possible. We created a chute using wooden panels on the sides and above the trailer. Then Kathy used her feminine side -- and marshmallows -- to lure Ben out of the trailer. After making it through the chute, the men flipped the huge steel cage on top of him. (The cage was like a box with no bottom.) Then the guys lifted the cage a few inches off the ground and walked along with Ben as he followed Kathy....or the marshmallows. To get over the small Jenni-made ponds, we removed the adorable little fence I had put up around them and laid several pieces of plywood over the entire area of water. Then Ben, the guys, and Kathy all scooted over the boards and toward the next gate. During this time I just held tight to my pole syringe with sweaty hands, hoping I wouldn't need to subdue a crazed animal.

They all took time to rest, then went several yards to the next gate. The entire time I was breathing a huge sigh of relief for each moment Ben was behaving. Then they passed the next gate, and proceeded down the hill. Finally, we were all in front of the pen. The coyotes were nowhere to be seen, as is always the case when we have a lot of strangers visiting the enclosure.

Again we made a chute, flipped up the cage, and in walked Ben. I could feel a huge load lift off me and the whole group. It was a success. Ben ambled around until he discovered something he had not had in more than a decade, a bathtub of water. It was actually a big bowl of water meant for drinking, but Ben had other plans. He looked ecstatic as he got in and set his entire butt into it. It had been a long hot trip in the trailer. Sitting there, he seemed to let all that stress out.

But there was more for him to discover. He had a *real* tub made from a huge cattle water tank! He made his way over to it, but didn't know what to do at first. After sniffing hesitantly, slowly and gingerly he got inside. Then he snapped and went crazy (in a good way)! He started swatting at the water, splashing and splooshing. All of us were happy for the show. We were thrilled for him.

I don't know how long he sat in his tub, but eventually he started exploring the pen, taking a bite of anything that seemed unfamiliar to him. Ben's next week guaranteed a new experience every day.

Ben pretty much ignored the two coyotes, Minnie and Scoopie, for the first several weeks, until Scoopie started getting bored with tormenting her sister and began biting Ben's butt from time to time while he ate. The first time I saw this, I was on our deck overlooking the backyard and Ben's new enclosure. I looked up to see Ben turn from his food bowl and glare at Scoopie, who was frisking about behind him. At the time I wasn't sure what had happened, but did see what had triggered his behavior a few days later, when I witnessed her biting his butt while he ate. Ben again exhaled loudly, giving her the stink-eye. She ran off. This happened several times within the first month, but tapered off after that. I suspect Ben smacked her or bit at her, or Scoopie just got bored with bothering him. She never did get sick of attacking her poor little sister though.

A very special event for us all was Ben's first ascension of the two-story tree house about a week after arrival. A staircase leads up to a 6 x 6 foot platform about 8 feet off the ground which has a smaller flight of stairs going another 4 feet higher to another platform which is built around an enormous tree. Torben lured Ben up the stairs with treats as the coyotes watched curiously. From then on, in the early summer mornings, you could always find Ben lying on the top platform, flat on his back with his legs spread out, usually with one of his back ones propped up against the tree. When lying like this, he was absolutely subdued, and that is when we began touching his head without needing to have food to distract him. We would stand on the lower platform while rubbing the enormous noggin that lay on the higher platform.

It would be several months before I felt I knew him well enough to pet him while he ate or was lying on his back. For the first 3 years it frustrated both me and Ben that periodically he would just want to follow me around. I never liked that because I never knew why he followed me. Though he was just like a big 400 lb dog in appearance, I didn't forget he was a bear.

A few years after Ben arrived, we built a new house on our acreage. After we moved; we were far away from Ben for several months because we had yet to build a new enclosure for him and the coyotes. I had several months to think about its dimensions and materials, and had it professionally built for a small fortune.

We now had to figure out how to move Ben yet again. We could recruit Kathy and Danny one more time for the short transport to the new enclosure. It seemed like a lot to ask of them since they each live far north of us, and the move with the bear would not even be a quarter mile by road. The real problem was still going to be just how we would get him up that same hill we so carefully had to take him down just a few years earlier on Mother's Day, surrounded by a large cage, held up by several devoted volunteers.

I got to thinking of all of Ben's new fans. Many would love to help move him to his new home. It makes for a good YouTube video too, especially if something goes wrong. Was it crazy to think we could move him all the way to the new pen the same way we had moved him the first time? As the crow flies, it is several hundred yards from one pen to the other, a very hilly few hundred yards, through several 5 foot wide gates. After much agonizing we decided our Plan A was to have him walk over while people surrounded him with wooden panels.   Just moments before trying it, we chickened out and went with Plan B. We pulled out the old heavy steel cage Ben came with. Remember it is about 5 x 5 x 5 feet of heavy steel. We were putting a lot of faith in our friends. We tilted the open bottom of the pen facing Ben's gate and used two large wooden panels to create a chute for him to walk through as we lured him with marshmallows. He innocently walked out. Once close to the transport cage we gently dropped it over him. Then the fun started.

Imagine about seven people circling a pen with a huge black beer, all moving as one organism slowly up a grassy hill, scooting carefully through gates, down a hill, up another, then along a long rocky driveway. I really wish someone had taken videos, though we were determined to not goof this up. Once we got to the rocky drive I worried about poor Ben's feet. He was going slower, gingerly even. We stopped to rest for his and our sake, praising Ben for his wisdom in being easy on us. He was happy to be getting more than his usual allotment of marshmallows and baby carrots, so did not seem too bothered by the fact that he was engulfed by this human mass that acted as one unit.

Finally, with tired arms and sore backs, we clapped as Ben took his first steps into the new enclosure. He did not have his two story tree house, but did have two choices of bathtubs, fun contraptions and tires and barrels to play with, not to mention his favorite toy "Planky," a 2 x 6 about 6 feet long that made a great baton for Ben once in a while. The new pen is adjacent to the side of our new back yard, close to our house. This meant I was able to spend even more time with him, learning his habits and getting to watch what "toys" he played with (only Planky so far!) and how he carried out his enriched feeding (typically meals hung on branches in the small forest that is all his). My favorites are putting marshmallows or hot dogs on the ends of small tree branches, and smearing jam or honey on the tree trunks. Thanks to our chickens, I often have enough eggs to give him an egg hunt once in a while as well.

In my eagerness to get Ben moved over that late spring, I had yet to build his den. I had hoped to provide him with another double platform structure but trashed that idea when I learned how much lumber I would need, and realized how difficult it would be to sink posts into ground that was mostly clay soil and tree roots. It would have to be a modest abode.

Ben missed being up off the ground. Fortunately, he caught the attention of a new volunteer, Lily. Lily had experience with sun bears and orangutans and was one of the few people we allowed to come and go into Ben's enclosure. Lily recruited her husband to make a raised platform on which Ben could lie, keeping him off the ground. They spent a long hot Sunday working on it, but were rewarded knowing Ben immediately started using it.

As summer wore on, I had to think about Ben's sleeping situation for the winter. Again, because of all the surrounding tree roots, and the hard soil, I knew a super tall structure was not going to be possible. I was able to get 10 foot long posts put in using those metal "cheats" as I call them. They are pointed at one end, can be pounded into the ground, then the wooden posts mounted onto them. Though I feel I cheated using them, it still sucked pounding them in. Multiple times I would have it going in nice and straight, only to notice eventually that each hit with the hammer caused it to angle a bit, likely due to a tree root. Pulling it up and then replanting probably took as much time as it would have to drive to a rental place, rent a large auger, then dig all four post holes. I just like doing things the harder way. This is true.

The 10 x 10 foot raised platform I built about a foot off the ground also needed walls and a roof. I am boring you, so will not go into details about my actually getting all the material I needed for the entire thing into my Honda Odyssey. Yes, strangers in the Menards parking lot offered assistance to the relatively small woman (who thinks she is much larger than she is) who was adamant she really "liked the challenge" of trying to get 10 foot posts, 2 x 4s, and 8 foot plastic panels into her minivan. Chivalry is not dead. Or maybe they all wanted the chance to witness and video my attempts. None the less, I did it.

Loading was not even close to the toughest part of this endeavor. Once home, I had to measure and cut boards outside the enclosure, then bring them in. A circular saw and electricity would have been more fun than Ben could have imagined. If I cut a board wrong, back out of the pen I went, recut, then back in again. I was grateful Ben loved Planky so much he preferred to play with that over the wood I was working with. However, when I brought the long corrugated plastic panels in, he thought he had a new toy.

I can't tell you how quickly my attitude changed from being enamored with Ben's curiosity to being utterly tired of it, as I stood on the top of a step ladder, using a cordless drill to screw the panels onto the roof. He just loved grabbing the panels as I got them up onto the roof, then kept nibbling at my feet. Remember, I was still uncomfortable to do more than pet Ben. His curiosity about me was still worrisome. Let me tell you, by the second day of building his hut, I was totally done with his drooly, happy, worn-toothed bear bites on my feet and ankles. He never bit hard, and seemed to just want to satisfy himself that I was not going to run away from him. Eventually, he thankfully would get bored, sniff around any tools I had carelessly left on the ground, then hop into his tub or find Planky.

By the time I was finished, the hut was painted with whatever spare paint I had, and straw had been spread around in it for a bed. Ben had already begun sleeping in his new hut. He and I had spent so much time together, I no longer felt nervous around him. If he is in "a mood" I leave him be. But sometimes I'll let him chew on my leg or arm. Though I have fantasies about being like that guy on TV who raised and trained the famous grizzly bear for movies, and I do play around and hug Ben, I have decided not to be utterly dumb, I do remember he is a bear I have known for only 5 years of his almost 25 years of life. To be honest, the only time he has ever hurt me was when I once let him have my hand. He bit down gently, as far as he was concerned, and put his head down while looking up at my face. It was excruciating but I didn't want to alarm him. He just looked at me with his small innocent eyes while I said "Ben, Ben, Ben, Ben, ow, ow, ow, ow …." I even blew on his face. He let go, then just kept sniffing me.

For a moment, I wondered, as I often do, whether I could still do surgery if I was missing that finger. It is a sick game I play with myself. The last time I played it was after being bitten on the right index finger by a rattle snake. Back then, I analyzed the situation carefully since there was a huge chance of my loosing it. But hey, there will be more on that in another chapter.

Finding the Story

I was doing an especially difficult surgery on a not-so-typical animal one afternoon when I remembered it was time for me to write another Witty Kitties Inc. newsletter article. What would I have to write about? My mind went back and forth between the surgery and my need to come up with a story.

As I started the rather lengthy suturing job, I thought of one possibility: Though Witty Kitties had never taken in dogs; we recently made an exception for six dogs from a puppy mill about two hours north of here that shut down. We really couldn't resist, as there were about 300 dogs that needed a place to go in a very short period of time. The plan was to hold them as long as needed, socialize them, and then move them to the local municipal shelter for adoption as room became available. We took in a beautiful golden retriever, two adorable beagles, two gorgeous huskies, and a rambunctious malamute. When taking them in, I hoped it wasn't going to be a mistake. But, after spending a few mornings witnessing Pasado the Naughty Donkey (yes, that is his name) running back and forth in front of the long run that runs along our big shed, playing with and taunting the malamute, I thought "Hey, why don't I write about how we should change our name to "Witty Kitties and Dorky Doggies?" No. Funny, but no real story there (no offense, dog lovers).

I had to think of something else. *Suture.*

My back was getting sore, so I moved around a bit before resuming suturing. So now what? Well, almost two weeks ago, I took on three baby squirrels that were injured when a tree was sawed down in Muscatine, where I had been working every other Friday. One had a head injury and seemed a bit "off" neurologically, and another suffered a broken humerus. OK, that's a story.

It was fun having those little guys, all eventually thriving, scampering all over me, watching them twitch and squeak the way only a squirrel can. But that is what they do. They eat, sleep, pee, poop, squeak, and scamper. Until they are older and go outside, their repertoire is limited. That's the extent of that story.

So, what then? *Suture.*

I kept up with the surgery, making sure the "bites" my needle made were consistent, not too big, and not too small. I do some of my best thinking during the routine portion of surgeries. Usually suturing large areas is very routine.

Next I wondered, what about the reptiles? I had just finished digging a new pond for Lex the Alligator but remembered Lex had had a lot of press recently. We had acquired him from a young man who had him for 5 years, keeping him in a kiddie pool in his basement while living in Iowa City. Though it was illegal for him to have such a pet within city limits, he was not giving Lex up for that reason, but rather because he was moving out of state and could not take him. Lex's first year with us was special. He was a topic of many conversations and had already been in the newsletter. No point in overdoing it.

I continued suturing, wondering what the heck was I going to write about? My back and neck and legs were getting really sore. Surgery was almost done. It had been the most difficult procedure I'd done up to that point in my career, but not because it was technically difficult. The challenge was that the entire surgery had been performed while I had been cramped in a fairly dark space of about 3 x 3 x 6 feet!

Yes, I was doing surgery in what was essentially a wooden box, the little insulated hut Amy and Roscoe, two of the pot-bellied pigs we had at the time, slept in. It was stinky and dusty and dark. What was I doing surgery on you may ask? I was doing surgery on Amy, the 150 pound pot-bellied pig's bum. Only minutes prior to putting her under on the spur of the moment, I noticed she had (okay, this is gross, but maybe that is what it takes to make my story interesting) a prolapsed rectum. What's that? Well, pretend you have a long stocking that is open at both ends. Put your hand half-way inside and pull the middle part of the sock out of the hole your arm is in. That inside part of the sock is what was sticking out of Amy. Actually, several inches worth of a very red, sore, and dirty "sock" were sticking out.

When I discovered Amy's problem I was home alone at about 3 in the afternoon on a spring day. Little Kirsten was in kindergarten and due home on the bus in less than an hour, and Joseph an hour after that.

Torben? God knew when he would be home as it was a Monday, a bad day for rural US postal carriers. I couldn't move Amy alone. She was taking up the back half of the 3 x 3 x 6 foot shack, stuck tight in the corner and not willing to move. I couldn't physically get behind her to push her out, and grabbing and pulling only elicited screams. Even if I had been able to get her out, we would have been out in the open for neighbors to see. Believe me, people felt if any weird animal thing was going on in our yard, it was time to come over and talk to us as though we enjoyed being the circus freaks I know they thought us to be. I had to repair her where she lay. No amount of cajoling worked either. Telling her that her life may depend on it fell onto deaf pig ears. She had declared where she wanted to be and no amount of coercion or bribery would work.

The day wouldn't stay light forever, so I had precious little time to get going. I hoped I could push the prolapsed rectum back in while Amy was heavily sedated. After getting her sleepy enough, while kneeling inside the shack, I tried pushing the protruding stuff back in. But it was way too big and damaged from sticking out for what could have been up to 8 hours considering I had not seen her since feeding time that morning. It was too swollen, and considering Amy's proximity to the ground and her desire to lie around in dirt and mud and poop, it was pretty filthy.

Looking at my watch, I realized Kirsten was due off the bus any moment. Stinking of pig pee and poop and God knows what else, I took off my rubber gloves, crawled out of the hut, brushed off the straw and dirt, and went to stand out at the mailbox to greet my little girl as she got off the bus. Shortly after salutations, I fed Kirsten news she was starting to get used to, news that meant another animal was going to keep Mommy busy for a bit.

"Hi Sweetie. Um, bad news. Mommy **has** to finish a surgery on Amy the pig."

"No you don't," she instructed.

"Yes, I **have** to."

"I'm hungry."

"Yes, first I'll get you something to eat."

"I wanna snuggle. Why do you smell? You smell like poop!"

We kept up the banter until I got it into my little Kirsten's head that I wasn't going to be able to dote on her the way I always did the second she got off the bus. She continued to whine, following me as I cleaned myself up so I could fix her a snack. Growing tired of her complaining about something I wasn't especially excited about doing myself, I decided to counter her pleas with blunt facts.

"Kirsten," I said slowly "If I don't do surgery right now, Amy will **die**!"

Barely caring, she looked at me like I was ridiculous for thinking I could be in control of the situation.

Then I said "SpongeBob is on."

That did it, her favorite cartoon. She made straight for the living room where I immediately brought her a snack, then turned on TV. She gave me the old heave ho by saying, "You're in my way," while I was standing in front of the TV, pointing the remote at it, adjusting the volume.

Back to Amy. Because the simple replacement of the prolapse had failed, she needed surgery. I had to give Amy more anesthetic. I tried again to pull her out of the hut, but the narrow space and her weight were too much. I had hoped to get her closer to the door to the outside so I could use the isoflurane machine with the oxygen tank attached to it. Inhalant anesthesia would be safer, but it was not to be. So I went into the house again to gather a surgery pack, prep, blade, sutures, and several pairs of latex gloves. Kirsten was still happily watching cartoons.

Taking my last breath of fresh air for a while, I crawled back into the cave-like hut. I know everyone is dying to know the details of what that surgery entailed, but I don't know if keeping your attention is worth that much grossness. Just know that I had to do an amputation of the portion of her rectum that was sticking out. Before cutting away the damaged tissue, it is important that the healthy portion it is attached to stays in place so it doesn't suddenly get sucked back into the body once the bad tissue is gone. This is done by putting "stay sutures" into the healthy tissue before cutting it 360 degrees. By the time I put the stay sutures in, Kirsten had come to the back door to ask if I was done.....for the first of at least a dozen times, each time forcing me to crawl on my hands and knees out of the box just to be able to hear her (the hut was well insulated). After responding to her, I would then crawl back into my box, don new gloves, and resume surgery. I was feeling guilty on so many levels and very taxed.

I was once again getting into my groove, kneeling and bent over due to the 3 foot ceiling, when I suddenly heard, "Mom! What are you doing in there?"

It was Joseph. I hadn't heard him drive home from school. After not finding me in the house, he asked Kirsten where I was. I can only imagine what she said. "She is in the pig house doing surgery on Amy's butt."

Answering him I said, "Um, I'll tell you later. Trust me, I would rather not be in here." I then added, "Could you watch Kirsten for me?"

I was half done with the suturing, and suffering from back spasms that had me cussing up a storm. I was glad my yelling was muffled by the walls of the hut. Finally, I couldn't take the backache and decided to lie on my stomach and elbows for the last of the suturing. So, Imagine walking up to my house, glancing over to the back yard, and seeing legs sticking out of a little pig hut, and periodically hearing !@#$%^&*! I was literally face-to-butt with Amy and hoping to God she would not have the sudden need to pee. (Pooping wasn't an issue since I had packed her rectum with gauze in the beginning. See? Told you this was gross!)

Compounding my discomfort and frustration was the periodic pecking at my feet by the two adult emus. Anything out of the ordinary was theirs for the pecking. My shoe laces fascinated them. They seemed convinced the laces should be theirs!

Towards the end of this nightmare, I realized Kirsten had dance practice tonight. I quickly shimmied my way out of the hut, feet first, on my belly. After slowly standing, I yelled into the house for Joseph to call Torben to see if he was on his way home from work, because I needed him to take Kirsten to dance practice. Joseph's driving permit did not allow him to drive anywhere but to and from his school when not with an adult.

Minutes later, I heard Torben pull into the driveway. He would have no time to eat a dinner if he wanted to get Kirsten to practice on time. Shimmying my way out of the hut feet first again, I saw Torben at the front gate with an expression that indicated he was not at all phased by the fact that his 40 something year old wife had just come out of a hut that was not much bigger than a large doghouse. And she was covered in shit. He then headed into the house and back out again with the little dancer and her dance supplies.

So, as I lay there alone to finish poor Amy's surgery, I looked around my cramped little space where I had spent most of the last three hours. Roscoe, the male pig, arrived at the opening of the hut and was telling me it was bed time. I turned my head to see him pacing with an annoyed look, threatening to step in, only to have my legs kick at him. I wasn't certain I'd survive him forcing his way through the door and walking on top of me, as he was nearly 200 pounds.

By the time I gathered instruments, needles and suture, dirty gauze, gloves, and the disgusting looking body part I had taken off of Amy, she was awake enough for me to leave. Roscoe was squealing at the top of his lungs to be allowed into his hut to be with his woman. I stepped aside and he wasted no time crawling in, mumbling something to himself. I couldn't understand it but am sure it was not nice.

I smelled like pig poo and was filthy. I had no time for my family all evening. I had forced my husband to skip dinner after a long day of work, and had ignored Kirsten and Joseph. The cloud of the old insanity seemed to be hovering again, which wasn't good. Later, as I scoured off the dirt and smell, and felt the deep muscle ache and tension, the grey cloud began showing its silver lining: I had my story.

The Carnivore's (Carnivore Keeper's) Dilemma

"I really wish snakes ate hotdogs. Then it wouldn't be so gross having them."

I remember agreeing with my friend and vet assistant many years ago, saying, "Yeah, then it wouldn't be so sad to have them."

We had just finished watching Torben leave the room where I kept our mice. Holding two of them in his hand cupped against his chest, he headed for the reptile room. He usually fed the snakes thawed frozen mice we ordered through the mail from a company that raises them for just that purpose. But once in a while we would take in a snake not used to eating already dead mice or rats. Until the snake could be "trained" to do so, it had to be fed live ones.

Just writing that sentence makes me sad.

You see, I am an absolute sucker for cute, fuzzy little animals. I actually have had little, fuzzy animals as pets for most of my life. I even went so far as to sneak my gerbils into the dorm my second year of college. I love snakes as well, finding them extremely beautiful and fascinating to watch. A big plus, too, is that compared to other domestic pets, you don't have to worry about "behavioral problems" like you may with dogs or cats. For example, if you get a sweet, roly-poly yellow lab mixed with whatever breed you want, (or not), you can hope he is as cool and smart as his dad or mom is; but you never know for sure in the beginning. He could be the odd lab mix that ends up being an obsessive-compulsive chewer, or barks at every noise, or never quite learns not to eat his own poop. Even with good training, a problem dog just may always be in need of correction or close supervision. You get my point.

With a snake, you pretty much know how it is going to behave from the day it is born or hatched (yes, some are born alive, some hatch from eggs), all the way well into old age. Snakes want very little in life; periodic meals, a spot to be warm and a spot to be cooler, water, and that is about it. If given those basic needs, snakes in general will behave in a predictable manner based on breed. The typical snakes we get are almost always constrictors who will bite when very hungry or not feeling great before a shed (because they literally shed the transparent skin on their eyes, they are temporarily blind, as the skin becomes opaque before peeling off). Certain species of snakes are known to be aggressive, such as the African rock python, which is to this day the one snake that requires a minimum of two people to control it: one person to hold behind its head, and the other to continually unwrap the snake's coils from around the person holding it.

Uh oh, soapbox time.

Let me just go off on a tangent before continuing on about the dietary requirements of snakes.

You remember the auction I mentioned back in the chapter, "In the Beginning"? Well the auction house didn't really care about who was selling what, or what type of care the animal was getting. It was and will always be money that persuades people to buy and sell animals as inanimate objects without any regard for the fact that they are sentient beings. To make matters worse, the sellers also don't care about whether the people buying the animals know what they are doing.

In spring 2006, a' guy called wanting to "get rid of a snake." What kind? A ball python," he said. OK, great, those are easy, not very big, and typically get adopted quickly. The man bought the snake at the wretched auction in April. Remember, we live in Iowa, so that can be a cold time. The man came with a very large Rubbermaid container. "Wow," I remember saying, "nice big container," assuming the guy just wanted a lot of space for the little guy. But when he picked the container up out of his vehicle, I could tell he put a little effort into it. Saying nothing, I led him to the reptile house, which at that time was still in our two-car garage.

He set the container down and I casually opened it. Oh my God, it was NOT a ball python! I did not know WHAT type of snake it was, but it was already over 5 feet long. "You said this is a ball python?" I asked. "Yea, I bought it this weekend. I never had a snake before and was told this is a good one to get." I bent down to take the snake out before realizing I didn't have a cage ready that would be big enough for it. I was expecting a ball python, something that doesn't get even close to 5 feet long.

"I got the snake home, but after a while it was moving around a lot more. My wife wouldn't let me take it out of the box," He said.

Once I put together a bigger cage, which was one that sat about face level with me, the now slightly warmer snake was indeed moving around. I managed to put it into the cage, closed it up, and waited for Torben to get home to tell me what the heck it was.

By the time Torben arrived home from work, I was eager for him to see the new "ball python." We went out to the garage. The cage was dark inside so he really couldn't get a good idea what was inside until he unlatched the cage door and opened it.

OUT shot the snake's head, barely missing Torben. It struck again, but Torben was ready for it this time. He grabbed it, putting one hand behind its head (something that takes two hands to do now, ten years later) and one along the snake's body, which was quickly wrapping around Torben's arm. "Oh my God, this is an African rock python. Get my arm, would ya?" I uncoiled the beast from Torben's arm and then helped hoist it back into its cage. I noticed, as he latched the cage back up, Torben was able to use only the one hand since the other had already turned a greyish blue color.

"Where'd this guy get that snake?" Torben asked. I then went into the long story about the auction, the evils of it, the evils of the people selling animals there, and the unsuspecting buyers, etc.....It wasn't until I finished telling him that I realized how lucky I was that I had not taken longer to set up the snake's cage. Any more time and it would have been plenty warm to lash out at me; and I didn't have the experience Torben had with handling such snakes.

So, today's soapbox take-home messages:

1. *Buying snakes is dumb, especially if you don't know what kind they are.*
2. *Auctions that sell pets are evil.*

Oh yea, snakes eat fuzzy, cute creatures. I love both snakes and fuzzy, cute creatures.

Danielle had pointed out that she wouldn't want a snake because "I like animals too much."

"Yeah," I agreed, not noticing my lack of consideration towards the poor snakes.

Months after this conversation, (but years before the African rock python came in), as Torben became known as "That Reptile Guy," taking various reptiles that'd come to us out into the community for special events and education, I found myself caring for dozens of snakes. I didn't think the feeding was so gross because I didn't have to take part in the killing of all those little mice and rats and bunnies. That problem was solved by a company far, far away from me. *Rodents R Us* (made up obviously) raises them in little plastic boxes equipped with food, water, bedding, and nothing else. The company sold them in a variety of sizes. For mice and rats it was "pinkies" (newborns), "fuzzies, hoppers, small adult, medium adult, XL adult," "XXL adult." or "XXXL adult." You can also select whether you want black or white haired mice, or even hairless, for those snakes who hack up hairballs.

Concerned about how the company killed the animals, I made a phone call and was told they used a virtually odorless carbon monoxide. This method is still used in labs and even at the occasional shelter. Knowing the poor things were not being put live into a freezer, I then started obsessing about how sad the rodents and rabbits must be, living without the stimulation of toys and a large environment. Contrary to what people think, rabbits are especially prone to boredom and need toys to chew, push around, and tunnel through. When I look at my own pet rat and mice, I take joy in seeing them on the wheels or climbing the variety of branches I've given them. The problem with providing an enriched environment, though, is that cleaning is a pain in the backside. This is no doubt why the feeder company does not do it.

So after being humanely killed, then packed nicely into insulated boxes of dry ice, they arrive at our door for a nice hefty price. How clean! How convenient! We warm them up and pop 'em into those hungry reptilian mouths. Just like hotdogs. Neat and bloodless.

A note here: you can't make snakes vegetarians. I could feed my family soy-based food products, but can't do the same for the snakes. I know this because once, in a fit of compassion for the rodents and rabbits who had probably had sad and boring lives, only to be killed in whatever mysterious way and shipped out as someone else's food, I did some research. As a result of my negative findings, I turned once again to possibilities for at least creating some sort of rodent/rabbit quality of life before their ultimate end. Ah! Anthropomorphism police take note. Though tiny little brains they may have, isn't a meager amount of enrichment justifiable, if not deserved? Happy mice. Happy food. Right? So, I decided to raise them myself.

My friends and Torben can tell you that over the years I've tried to do this on and off many times. I'd start and then stop due to lack of time to keep the cages (and all those enriching toys) clean, or I couldn't keep up with the demand. Then too, sometimes the witty kitties would figure out how to get into the cage, or (and this is often) I'd start holding a mouse or rat and decide I liked it too much, or (sound the sirens, anthropomorphism police!) it "liked" being held and "wanted" to be my pet. Try as I could, I'd always give up raising "feeder" animals. I truly believe "happy" mice, or rats, or anything for that matter, should somehow mean healthier and, therefore, better food. I also like the thought of decreasing the numbers of animals run through the feeder company.

The following spring we discovered the mysterious arrival of baby bunnies running around in the yard of our old farmhouse the day after Easter, I had never made an attempt to do the same with bunnies. The bunnies that showed up were likely rejects from someone trying to sell "Easter Bunnies" to the public. It wasn't long before they became 18 rabbits running around in our fenced in yard. Of course eventually they figured out how to leave the yard. I often heard cars honking at them on the road, or neighbors yelling something like, "Hey! Your damned rabbit is out!" I'd yell back, "It's mine only by default! Leave me alone!" I was catching and neutering as fast as I could, but obviously it was not fast enough. Once I accepted that we had a **lot** of rabbits, most of which were not at all easy to handle and so could not be adopted out as pets, I quit neutering them and began keeping a small population as reptile food. I kept them in a big enclosure with grass and sunshine. They ran around and played. I was glad that they were "happy." Happy food. Yeah, that's right.

Then they had babies, such cute babies! It was immediately obvious my venture would fail, just as it had with the rats and mice. Providing rabbits as food didn't last beyond the one generation. I didn't quit raising them because I thought it was wrong. Nor did it make me too sad. No, I quit when a neighbor man made a special trip to tour our shelter with his children and said, "Hey, I know someone who might want two rabbits for pets. That way you won't have to kill them." He seemed to have a scornful look on his face. I got it, I was a bad person. It didn't matter to the guy that these rabbits served multiple important purposes. Did he mean we should starve the snakes? Should some sad bunnies a thousand miles away deserve to live a boring life only to be killed? I couldn't begin to explain the complexities.

It was then that I really experienced the dilemma. Torben deals with people like that man all the time. "Why do you have to KILL things to feed the snakes?" I had always known how passionate Torben is about reptiles, especially snakes. Anyone who knows him knows that. And I always thought I understood it. Of course I would think I got it. I love animals. Reptiles are animals, hence..... Say no more.

But it wasn't until recent years that I *really* started to understand the *why* of his passion. It hadn't occurred to me that my love for turtles, tortoises, geckos, etc., didn't mean I was embracing **all** reptiles. Snakes had always been a fascination for me, but the love took time. You don't really "bond" with snakes. Snakes are hairless, can't come when called (no ears!); there is no whining when hurt, or purring when content. They also don't have facial expressions to read. Heck, they look the same sleeping as they do awake! Remember the whole thing about shedding the skin on their eyes? Well that skin is essentially the eyelids which are fused right to the eye. The eyes don't move, but are just sort of a continuation of skin. Yet, I must admit there is something extraordinary about snakes. And...they must eat.

Now let me tell you how this dilemma gets even *more* complicated. Frequently, rabbits, rats, or other rodents are brought into animal control facilities for whatever reason. And, many times, they are not good candidates for adoption (aggression and biting are common reasons) or the shelter is overrun by rabbits at the time. What do you do with that animal? I can tell you I've taken several home, neutered them, and let them run on my farm. But what else can be done with them? They are euthanized by lethal injection, put into a freezer, and then picked up by a service that cremates them. You might be seeing where this is headed.

Only recently, I diagnosed probable uterine cancer in an older female rabbit at a local shelter. She was 7 or 8, and not the most adoptable compared to the tame little butterballs the shelter already had. She was euthanized peacefully and disposed of. I think that was a waste of a rabbit. I think it was a waste of a body. I say that at the risk of getting many haters out there. (Get in line people!) That rabbit could have been a month's worth of meals for a large snake, thereby reducing the number of sad-life feeder rabbits by one. Of course, the shelter was *not* going to risk a rumor or bad press. Most of the public generally accepts (though not all) that lethal injection is the preferred form of euthanasia. Nice and neat.

"Jenni, you mean to say you want to feed people's former pets to snakes? That is so cruel!" I can hear the chorus.

Of course not. I can imagine what a public relations nightmare that would be. But would it? Only recently have I come to grips with the practicality. Before you tune me out and toss this book into the nearest garbage can, I want to make an extremely important point about how an animal dies when killed by constrictors, the type of snakes we have. (Other ways snakes eat: kill with venom, then eat; or eat the still-living prey.) Constricting snakes kill *quickly* (recall how quickly Torben's arm went blue and numb?) and prey do not suffocate from being squeezed so hard. In recent years it was discovered (using fluoroscopy I believe) that the constriction is so quick and strong that it literally collapses blood vessels and the heart stops. Shock, and then fainting, is what the prey feels. Of course, for huge prey, like antelope or people (according those who have escaped it), it is not so quick. But we are talking small, easily-constricted, easily-swallowed prey. It is very fast. I'm beginning to sound like Torben now — "prey," "constriction," "Snakes Rock, Man!"...

Do I watch live prey feeding? No. I still favor fuzzy animals over scaled ones. Even though I still don't have that deep, deep, deep, passion for them, that my husband does, I do want them to eat. What is best for the animal in our care may not be seen as appropriate by the public. But we must let the public know that we have carnivores. *Carnivores by nature, not choice*. This whole eating meat thing stinks in a way, but what do you do? You can say all you want that "People shouldn't have those big snakes anyway." Well, no duh. But the snakes continue to come to us, and we must provide them with food, water, and shelter. With the fairly new laws in Iowa, we hope fewer and fewer people will feel compelled to buy snakes that get to be over 20 feet long.

So, I love fuzzy little animals. I love snakes. This is my dilemma.

(BTW, snakes don't hack up hairballs. Hair comes out in their poop.)

Frenemies: Leave Your Offerings to the Raccoons

"No good deed is left unpunished."

That's the truth.

I find myself wondering why I do things I feel are "nice" at the time, only to have them bite me in the butt later. The "nice" thing I have in mind is the rehabilitation Torben and I did of so many baby raccoons back in year 3 or 4 BK (Before Kirsten). I've told stories in the past detailing the fun of having hungry baby coons crawl up my bare legs to get their food, taking some on a camping trip in the VW van, and discovering one knew how to flush the toilet. I think those same raccoons (more likely their offspring's offspring) are returning the favor in their special way. They seem to see the house as a place where the free food will continue forever. "Hey, Jenni! You did such a great job. Look what we can do!"

The last summer when we lived in the old farm house, I had a big fat red hen and two white silkie hens. They shared a big nest with about a dozen eggs in a hutch right off the side of our back deck (next to the hut I sat in while doing surgery on Amy's butt). If you think chickens are a boring subject, you just have not met the right chicken. They are actually quite clever, trainable, and seem to have very distinct personalities. Also they are just stinking cute! If you don't know what a silkie chicken is, imagine a small bird with snow-white Angora rabbit fur all over its body, causing it to look three times bigger than it really is. Adorable!

These chickens were also diligent in keeping the eggs warm, and very protective of the clutch. When a duck or another of our dozen or so chickens came by, the hen stationed at the nest (sometimes two or even all three at a time) would ruffle up her feathers, lean forward with her tail tilted forward, and make a noise I liken to an angry Chihuahua growling while under a big pillow. One morning while doing chores, I noticed no hens were on the nest, and no eggs were in it. I thought maybe Torben had taken the eggs to feed to the coyotes or bear, thus causing the hens to leave. Not something I would have expected Torben to do, but with all the possibilities, this was the best scenario.

It was minutes later when I discovered a wing from the big fat hen in the yard. A few bloody white fluffs scattered about were all that was left of the silkies. The most likely culprits? Those naughty raccoon offspring. I was pretty peeved because I love my hens and fresh eggs. I was also annoyed because we had over 30 Muscovy ducks in nests all around the yard, reproducing like rabbits, and none of them had been touched. I don't wish ill on my ducks; but if a bird from my yard has to go, I'd rather it be one the dozens of ducks than my few favorite chickens.

The next few nights were fine. Some of the remaining chickens roosted on our deck just outside the sunroom, the others in a large pen I could close them into easily.

But raccoons are awfully brave. A few mornings later I noticed new bits and pieces of evidence. Scattered about the yard were parts of another hen. I looked around and of course came up short on my head count. I also noticed all the eggs from another nest, this time a duck's, in our front yard were gone.

I picked up the remaining chickens off the deck railings to lock up with the others, and reinforced the pen of a new bunny I had just taken in. Everyone had to be penned up as safe as possible. As I did this I had to be aware of the male emu, Schoonie, who at that time of year was completely out to get me. I was the main human who fed and cared for him and his female partner, Flynnie. I was also the only human he consistently attacked; pecking and high kicks became his daily workout. If I raised my hands and stood up tall he usually backed off. It worked better, though, if I had something in my hands to make me seem even bigger. Often at that time of year, neighbors could see me with a pail or two in my hands, holding them high or waving them at the enormous bird. But when the "something" in my hands happened to be a live chicken or rabbit, I instead held the poor critter to my chest and walked with my back towards Schoonie. Sometimes this ended without incident and other times it ended with a forceful thump to my back side. It was a chore making sure he was distracted while I made the repeated trips from the house to the pen. He was a very unappreciative bird, over 100 pounds, with a brain not much bigger than a chicken's.

I asked Schoonie, while he struck and hissed at me, "Where were you when my chickens were getting slaughtered at night?!" A watch-emu he was not.

The raccoons harassed me in other, non-fatal ways as well. As a matter of fact, I can say with complete honesty that the raccoons even went so far as to take Jesus away from me. Yes, the raccoons stole my baby Jesus, literally. You see, I used to have a really lovely Nativity scene I was quite proud of. It was a classic, hand-painted, ceramic collection: Mary, Joseph, kings, camel, angel, etc. Though I do not practice the Catholic religion I had been raised in, I did find great joy in setting up the scene each winter. Jesus first, then I'd place the entourage around him, trying to create a unique scene each year.

After Christmas, I gently placed each figurine into the special-shaped holes in the thick rectangular piece of packing foam they came in. Once in their respective spots, I put the foam piece into its original box and stored it in the loft of our big shed. Along with the Nativity set box, I had at least four big tubs of decorations that were stacked in the same area.

One day during the summer I had to go up into the loft to retrieve some cages we also stored up there. As usual, I had to step over a sizable pile of raccoon poop at the top of the steps, then stumble over crates and cages that had been neatly stacked at one time, but had been knocked over by the nocturnal beasts who seemed to think nothing was off limits to their curiosity. When I got close to the area where the Christmas boxes were stored, I noticed chunks of packing foam on the floor. I didn't think a lot about it until I found a head. It belonged to one of the three kings. Suddenly aware of the source of the foam pieces, I hurried to the Christmas boxes, where I discovered the entire Nativity set box had been torn to shreds. I immediately began picking up body parts, Mary's top half, Joseph's bottom, a donkey's ear. I searched and collected until I could account for everyone in the group, or at least a portion of everyone in the group, with one exception. Jesus was missing.

The loft is in the center of our huge shed and overlooks the two halves of the building. Many pieces of the set had fallen to the back, lesser-used, darker portion of the shed. I had not replaced the burned out bulbs on the ceiling because the light fixtures are about twenty feet off the ground, so I searched for Jesus with my flashlight. As I hunted, I found myself making up, then humming, a song in my head. It had a country melody and went something like "Oh, here I am.......in the dark......my light in hand....looking for my Jeeeeesus." It was actually quite good, and made me laugh. But it did not help in finding my baby boy.

Defeated, I gathered up what I could, including the now-empty crib, and took them to the house. I felt an attachment to them, so I refused to throw them away.

111

They sat around for years before one day I decided to showcase them. There was no way I could piece them all together, so I chose to use them in a mosaic on the wall at the base of the small porch of our old farmhouse. I didn't think it was sacrilegious for two reasons: I wasn't the one who broke them, and I didn't put them in any sort of compromising arrangement. All in all, I think the entire wall looked very nice, my Nativity pieces placed at random with broken plates, cups, and glasses. I almost wish I still had that wall here at the new house. Sadly, the process of putting them onto the concrete wall permanently made it impossible to salvage them before demolition of the house.

The raccoons also harassed me in the more traditional way by breaking into our animal feed. I marvel at how a 15 pound slab of limestone on top of a flat garbage can is no deterrent for those little rascals. Bungee? Lame. Plastic bins? Say goodbye to those. Raccoons have chewed through so many tubs trying to get into the feed that I have a collection of at least a dozen huge bins with no tops.

Many folks would say, "Why not trap the raccoons and release them elsewhere? Or shoot them?" I don't feel right about that. They tick me off when they get into our feed, poop in our sheds, and eat my other animals. I think if you live in the country, even in a residential area in the country, you should expect animals as part of the package. I was slow in finally realizing the solution was that I had to put more effort into ensuring the rest of my prey animals are safe at night. It is a nuisance, but not very difficult.

Soapbox: People who go to extremes to rid their area of possums and raccoons are the same ones who pollute their yards with chemical fertilizer and herbicide. If you live in the country, what is wrong with letting your yard consist of whatever natural ground cover comes along? I happen to like dandelions, wild violets, and creeping charlie. If I wanted my yard to look artificially perfect, I would live on a golf course.

Some people really go to extremes to "win" over nature despite wanting to live out in the country. I have a disturbing story about a man I met at the front desk of a pet store. A friend of mine owned the store, and he was one of her suppliers. My friend was in the back checking on her inventory, while he and I stood near the register at the front of the store. which had a large picture window looking into the parking lot where my 24 ft long veterinary unit was parked. From the inside of the store I could see one of the raccoons I had at the time was up on the dashboard pacing back and forth, probably putting pencils and pens down into that crack between the dashboard and windshield. I am certain the little guy knew it was impossible to get them out once down there. So this supplier decided to tell me about a difficult raccoon he dealt with the previous summer. He laughed as he told it. When I asked him if the story was going to get ugly he chuckled "Oh, no. This is great. You'll see." I had made it clear to him that I **liked** raccoons, but don't think he would have gotten that into his thick skull if I had hammered it in.

I listened patiently to the man's story, once in a while looking towards the back of the store for my friend. Where was she? He went on about how no matter what he did, he could not keep the raccoon out of his garbage can. Bungee cords and bricks on the lid were kids-play for that raccoon.   The man continued, "But then I finally caught the raccoon **in** the garbage can!" He had a sparkle in his eye that made me feel uneasy as he said, "I dragged that garbage can to the middle of the street, and then got the gas can...."

(Note: Due to its graphic nature, the squeamish may want to skip the next paragraph to avoid images that will haunt you and raise your blood pressure.)

The story finally ended with the raccoon engulfed in flames, running back into the man's garage, going into the rafters, and setting it on fire. He thought it was hilarious. "See? Isn't it crazy?" said the man I now hated.   "The raccoon ended up winning! My garage was in ruins! I told you it was a great story!"

Ha Ha.

When my friend returned to the front, I am sure my face was pale. She sent him on his way, then apologized for the man. I told her to never again allow me in her store if he was there.

I am a far cry from that "man." Despite the cussing I do each time the raccoons take the lid off the livestock feed, or even kill one of my birds, it just shows that we must have done a great job at raising the little raccoons and releasing them into the wild. They thrived well enough to multiply and I guess they're back coming to show off their hunting skills is their way of saying "Thanks." Yet if I want to deter them, it doesn't hurt to leave the raccoons an offering of food each night at the shed and at our house. I find about three to five pounds of dog or cat food will do. (I know I'm feeding all those opossums I fostered as well.) And I thank the Lord for all the donations we receive.

in-ˈsa-nə-tē

I'm not so sure I agree with Albert Einstein's definition of "insanity," doing the same thing over and over again while expecting different results. When I first heard it many years ago it made sense. But since then I've found that nature throws so many variables into the equation that it is almost impossible to do the same thing exactly the same way as before.

I go more for those traditional definitions, "dementia, lunacy, madness, craziness, mania" and so forth. However, even those aren't necessarily a bad thing. I think some of the most fun, creative, effective things I've made in life were made during a period of certain madness. However, that is not to say my **worst** things were not made during times like that as well.

Here is an example of just one of many insane days I've experienced, one that doesn't involve a crazy animal chasing me, nor does it involve Torben getting bit by one (those fall into my humorous stories), nor does it involve an animal escaping or doing anything bizarre. No, animals are not the cause of the insanity. The only species I believe capable of true insanity is the human.

Kathy, the equine rescue goddess, often uses me as her veterinarian in abuse/neglect cases when the equine-specialists are not available. The scenarios are pretty routine. I look at the horses. If I feel they are showing signs of endangerment or neglect, I say so

116

and they are removed from the premises, with the assistance of law enforcement of course.

The two stallions in this story had a very low body score, and showed evidence of untreated injuries, especially of the limbs. Law enforcement and another veterinarian agreed on their deficiency in care. I wrote a report and submitted it. But, as is often the case, the owner contested it, meaning he pretty much disagreed his horses looked like crap. It never ceases to amaze me that the same people who do not spend a bit of time or money on feeding their own animals then use an incredible amount of time, money, and energy to get their animals back!

Insane.

I received the subpoena. Kathy and I drove off to one of quite a few cases like this. We drove two hours to (fill in the blank) county courthouse. It was, as are most old courthouses, huge, spacious, and beautiful. Admittedly, I still find them fascinating. The architecture, art, and history seem to be written all over them.

We went to the clerk's office to sign in and show our subpoenas. Oddly, though, the office was locked. That was something we hadn't seen before. A note on the door said that, due to budget cuts, the office would be open only on certain days and for shorter hours. We were there on the wrong day. The attorney on the case said not to worry, she'd take care of making sure our appearance was documented, and do whatever else the clerk's office would have done.

The courtroom was on the third floor. At least we had a nice view of the atrium from up there. It wasn't unusual to have to wait a while. So Kathy and I sat down on one of the long wooden benches that reminded me of church pews and chatted. We also people-watched, primarily the officers sitting on the bench about 20 feet from us. When we first arrived, there were four of them. Two were county deputies, one a jail officer, and I believe the other a patrolman. They were chatting, shooting the breeze, and obviously waiting for their own court cases to start.

We waited about an hour before the county's lawyer said she was still working on something. She asked Kathy for some advice. Since animal court cases were rare in this particular county, even the lawyers weren't up to speed on some of the logistics. Who would pay for the horses' care while under Kathy's care, for example? The lawyer went away.

I noticed there was another jail officer in the group near us by now. None of us had set foot into the courtroom yet.

Another hour went by. Two of the officers left without going into the room, and a new deputy arrived. I started calculating what they made hourly and how much it cost taxpayers for them to just sit there. Kathy and I whispered how nice it would be to get paid for sitting and waiting. They were. We were not.

The lawyer came back and said, "He (the defendant) wants the horses back." " Well no duh. That is why we are here, right?" I thought. She and Kathy talked. I kind of spaced out so don't know exactly what they were talking about. I just wanted to go in and testify so we could get out of there.

I tuned in to their conversation just as the lawyer said, "I'm having him (the defendant) come over to talk to you." Now that was unprecedented. Kathy seemed as bewildered as I was. But sure enough the man who had allowed three of his horses to starve, one to the point that it couldn't walk and had to be destroyed on the spot, was standing by us with his hand out. We both shook it. Why?

Insanity.

That is why. I have an ingrained need to be nice and don't have the courage to say. "No thank you, I don't shake the hand of animal abusers."

The guy gave the typical sob story of how his ex was to blame, and how the horses all "seemed fine a week ago", and on and on and on. Though I felt myself tuning out again, I did hear the words, "I've had horses most of my life." as though that meant he actually knew what he was doing. Based on my experience of having horses when I was younger, and not knowing a fraction of what I should have, this isn't always true. I knew so little, and for that my horses suffered in their own way. Just because you had or did something "all your life" does not mean you did it well.

He also wanted to breed them, despite the fact that the value of horses has dropped so significantly that people abandon them in pastures all over the state rather than keep them. Auction prices aren't even worth the cost of getting them to the auction. Breed already-unwanted animals?

Insane.

I'll cut to the chase. The lawyer let the guy have his horses. No court case. The guy was to pay Kathy for her care of the horses. He would pick them up on such and such a day.

We were at the end of our third hour in the court house when three of the officers who had been waiting went into their courtroom one at a time for a few minutes each. What the other officers were there for, I can only guess. But when we finally left, four officers were still in the hallway. "Wow, must be an important case," I thought. "But I'll bet it cost a whole lot of money to have them all there. Gee, the budget cuts must be working, right?"

Insane.

Kathy and I did some ranting and raving as we often do after something like this, regardless of how the case goes. We were both really peeved that we had been subpoenaed for a case that never happened. Our entire day was gone. Boy at least there will be sort of compensation from the county. Right?

A few days later, the horses were back in the man's possession. Two weeks hadn't gone by before I heard he was having difficulty being able to feed them. Surprise, surprise.

I griped about the whole thing for a few days, but let it go eventually. A real sock to the gut was when I opened an envelope from the county many days later. It was compensation for my entire day. The county could redeem itself by paying me at least something. They had no trouble paying multiple officers for doing nothing but stand around a court house.

Inside the envelope was a check for $5.00.

Insane.

Living a Cliché (The Snake Bite)

I know it is easy to grab onto images of what you think life should be, or to try living the life others think you should lead. It is a comfortable way to go, really. I know I followed my own preconceived images of what my life should be like for a long time. But I also struggled against them as well, feeling confined. As a result, I eventually started "winging it" in life, if you will. I'm not saying it is a smart way to go, just the way I seem to go.

One of my two favorite quotes is from the wonderful icon Sophia Loren, "Mistakes are part of the dues one pays for a full life." Sure, Ms. Loren isn't a famous politician, religious figure, or philosopher; but she has obviously led a full and meaningful life. And while she might point to some of her mistakes, surely she also seems to have gotten some of it "right."

Maybe this philosophy is why I seem to take on such odd challenges – following that old gut of mine instead of my brain – paying little or no mind to what common sense is screaming at me.

Maybe though, this is also what brought me to the events that taught me to give in and live this way. My life as a cliché. But I digress....

March 22, 2009 started out pretty normal. It was Sunday, raining, and chores were taking up most of our morning as usual. Someone stopped by to report four cats had been dumped at the end of the Witty Kitties drive-way. This was also a regular occurrence.

So, I walked over to the shelter's driveway, several hundred feet from ours, grumbling, angry at the people who were inconveniencing me on a morning most people would be relaxing. By the time I got to the crates and saw the frightened, huge eyes of the kitties, and heard their mewing, my sour mood turned to complete empathy for the sudden change these animals were having to experience. They had been house cats, all well into adulthood, and were now cold and huddled in crates that allowed the rain to drip in through the slats. It is because I can suddenly turn on the "caring for the animals," and turn off the "pissed as hell at whoever dumped these cats," that I am able to do what I do. This trait also keeps me mostly sane.

Checking the cats in meant doing a brief exam, weighing them, vaccinating them in case they weren't up to date, and finding a place for them in the Witty Kitty compound. It took a bit of time, a few hours. You have to remember, Witty Kitties is not an animal control agency; It's a limited-admittance shelter for special-needs cats and exotic animals. This fact is lost on many people, hence many animals are dumped here. By the time I was done, it was almost 3:00. There went my morning and early afternoon.

Little did I know just how interesting the rest of the afternoon was going to be. I stopped by the house to check on Joseph and little Kirsten, who were hanging out together in the living room. Then I joined Torben who was in with the reptiles.

Torben asked me to help with a new game he invented called "let's-take-the-sluggish-half-asleep-rattlesnakes-out-to-sex-them-before-they-are-too-rambunctious-to-handle-once-they-are-out-of-hibernation". Sexing reptiles isn't terribly easy. You need to probe their cloacae (the single opening they have down there, used for pooping, peeing, and sex). Why did we have rattlesnakes? The question *should* be, "Why did someone *else* have rattlesnakes?" The original owner was sent off to serve in Iraq. He left them in his apartment for his landlord to find. No warning.

You would not believe how many animals are simply left behind in the event of a move. Landlords I've met have found snakes, pet tarantulas, cats, and dogs. I once adopted an abandoned, tiny, long-haired Chihuahua, "Charlie Bear," who was bald and red due to demodectic mange. He, his mate, and daughter had survived alone in an apartment for 5 days before being found. Their only water was a pail of dirty mop-water containing some sort of cleaning chemical. Not sure they even tried drinking it, or could have reached into the pail. My point is, some people utterly and completely suck.

Whew, where was I? My snakebite story... I was talking about sexing rattlesnakes, I believe.

Now, my venomous snake-handling experience was not huge. I learned to catch water moccasins by watching Torben, and had managed to catch one the previous summer on a favorite snake road in southern Illinois. I had also casually picked up, with my bare hands, what I thought was a baby fox snake in the beam of our van's headlights one night, only to find out it was a pygmy rattlesnake. But handling venomous snakes wasn't a daily thing for me. So it was kind of exciting to help, and I was happy to add to my list of "weird" things I've done in this life. Yet I also noticed a bit of hesitancy at the task, which I felt was good. It would keep me careful.

Note: Before I continue, let me just say that Torben and I both know the proper process would have been to have the snake slither into a tube with a screen of some sort on the other end that would force it to stay put and be unable to turn around. Too smart for us at the time though.

We had just finished the first snake, Torben probing and me holding, when Torben told me to go ahead and put her into the empty plastic container that was waiting for her. I briefly hesitated; and almost asked if I needed to do anything in particular as I let her go, since we had just annoyed the heck out of this snake. (Prior to the procedure, you could casually pick up and handle them. After sexing them, they were very active.) Well, I leaned down to quickly release her, when she did that contorting thingy snakes do so well, and she curved part of her mouth back and just hooked my right index finger with a fang while I simultaneously dropped her into the container.

"I got bit," I said, or something like that. "What do I do?" Most people may think it odd that I ask this of a layperson, but Torben knows more about snake envenomations than anyone I know. My question was honest. Statistically, I should be fine, or maybe at worst, have a horrible localized reaction. At the *very* worst, maybe even lose a finger. That would not be too great, but I'd have to live with it. So I just found myself wondering if there was something I should do.

The bite was a tiny dot, yet bled very readily. And it *really* hurt. I washed it, then sat down at the kitchen table with an ice pack on it, feeling a great sense of sadness. I had disappointed someone. Me? Torben? The snake? By being bitten. I felt foolish. After a good ten minutes, during which I told Joseph I had been bitten but should be fine, I stood up once again to wash my hand which was still bleeding profusely (too much for so long after the bite). I immediately heard blood rushing in my ears and said, "Wow, I hear blood swooshing in my ears..." and passed out cold.

This is what I remember of those seconds of being out:

I saw a bright green background, and heard a little girl's laughter. It was coming from a little flying bird in front of me that suddenly became Kirsten. I was bewildered, then suddenly awakened, looking up at

Joseph who was gently slapping my face, saying "Mom! Mom!"

Torben called 911.

Thank goodness it took less than ten minutes for the paramedics to arrive. I was oddly calm, mellow, and very much okay with being on the kitchen floor as strangers slowly filed into our kitchen. I remember Cha Cha and Mumma, the dogs, wanting to hang out with me, and Trixie, our chubby cat who loves licking things, licking my hand obsessively. It all seemed fine with me at the time, though I'm sure it looked comical. I was just going with the flow, not realizing my calmness was likely due to my dropping blood pressure and therefore weakening oxygen supply to my brain.

Even though my blood pressure was low the first time the paramedic checked, and even lower the second time, the two (or three?) paramedics, a Johnson County cop, Torben, the pets...... were all pretty calm. JoJo had kept 4 year old Kirsten busy in the other room. I think she was not too upset by the scene because her brother, who proved to be more of a man than I could have ever imagined at 14, told her everything was just fine, and played with her.

Finally, I was lifted in a sling and carried down the stairs and out of the house. As I was being put into the ambulance, I suddenly felt I AM NOT OKAY. Prior to this moment, I just felt mellow, not weak, and just very calm. But now that feeling was gone. As we pulled away from the house the nausea started. It came on hard!

The paramedic, one of many people who provided multiple miracles that day, put an IV catheter into my arm. After the vomiting started, I realized she was putting in a second IV. My thoughts were, "Gee, must really need those fluids, I guess....." but still I believed this was not going to be too serious a problem.

The vomiting quickly became uncontrollable and violent. Each time I retched, my legs came up and my body curled tight. It was too much to think I'd manage not to pee in my pants at that point. Up until then I was pleased with myself for having on clean underwear for my trip to the hospital. I actually thought about those things.

At this point things started getting hazy. I could hear exchanges between the paramedic who was driving, and the paramedic who was in the back with me, trying to pump fluids into me, and simultaneously trying to calm my lurching body. Urgency was now apparent. Torben was in the passenger seat, trying to reassure me. I could also hear his conversation with the driver. He was startled by how many cars were not pulling over for an emergency vehicle on the freeway. "Why the hell don't these people pull over? Does this happen a lot? How do you handle it?" I imagined people lolly-gagging along the freeway down to Iowa City, not looking even once into their rearview mirrors at the flashing lights on their tail.

Suddenly, I experienced a sensation I'll never forget. It felt as though every single pore on my body opened and sweat simply started pouring out. I realized immediately I was going into shock. After that I only had on and off moments of blurred consciousness.

I remember hearing shouting and seeing dull visions as I was taken out of the ambulance. Then, the next moment I couldn't see anything, but was being yelled at by people I didn't even know. I couldn't figure out why they were so angry at me. "Who's slapping me?" I thought. I opened my eyes to a man's head over my face, silhouetted by the bright lights above us. "Jennifer! Jennifer!" "Jenni! Sweetie!" Emergency staff and Torben were shouting. "Open your eyes! Say something! Look at me! LOOK at ME!" I heard these words interspersed with some unnerving words I understood all too clearly. That is when I finally got scared.

I remember hearing I was in "a-fib" and that my blood pressure was "40 over not." I heard the words "We're losing her" and, worst of all, that I was "in DIC."

Let me explain DIC. Disseminated Intravascular Coagulation, also fondly known by doctors (of humans and animals) as "Death Is Coming," means that the blood in your vessels literally clots. As a result, the limited amount of clotting factors in the blood are depleted, hence allowing spontaneous hemorrhage from capillaries, causing unstoppable bleeding from a variety of orifices. As a veterinarian I had NEVER saved an animal in DIC, regardless of cause.

I continued to have the violent heaving, attempting to vomit. I heard someone order propofol, an IV anesthetic, and realized they needed me a bit anesthetized to get me to stop moving around. I felt two pairs of scissors cutting off my clothes, each starting at the front legs of my shorts. They simultaneously moved to my waist, then higher. I remember thinking at that moment, "Clean underwear?" Not anymore. "Hey, they cut my new pink bra and my Obama t-shirt! Will I get them back?"

It was shortly after these crazy thoughts that I had a profound realization. As I weakly turned my head to the doctor, who repeatedly insisted I keep my eyes open, I understood that I was dying.

Up until then, I felt this was going to pass over, as so many of my other injuries had. I thought then of nothing but my kids. I can't die! They couldn't not have a mom! The strongest force keeping me awake (or alive) was just how angry and haunted I knew Joseph would be if this were to be the way I died.

Joseph is very much like his father, my first husband. He always worries about my safety with the animals, as well as my difficulty taking care of myself when I have animals to care for first. While lying there, my verbatim thought was, "JoJo will be SO PISSED if I die this way!" He would live his life angry with me, knowing he had been right all along, knowing I was pushing myself too much, not worrying about the effect it was having on others. He knew my tendency for caring too little about me, and too much for the animals.

I do believe my hearing and understanding the medical terms that were implying my demise was not the curse some may think. It was very clear to me now that I was almost dead, and that knowledge actually caused me to concentrate on opening my eyes and staying awake.

There was a sharp pain in my groin on the right. I knew they were putting in a large bore IV catheter. I really needed blood pressure. I assume they must have given me the propofol then. I was fading out.

My next vague memories are of the following day, Monday. I was in a bright room, the ICU, with white towels around my head. There were bright red blood spots on those towels. I was still spitting up blood. I couldn't speak. I had a tracheal tube down my throat, yet I remember feeling strangely calm about not being able to speak or close my mouth.

Oddly, one of my first thoughts was that it was "March Madness" season. I felt bad that Torben had been hanging around, probably bored stiff. (I later found out he sat in my room the previous night, talking to me, and reading the sports section to me. It was probably the first time he did that without me interrupting him with a lame question. I don't like sports much). I noticed the TV in front of me. I tried communicating as best I could that he didn't have to just sit there. Eventually I wrote "Sweet 16" on a pad of paper he held for me, and motioned dribbling a basketball with my hand. Not sure when he got it, or if he did, but I think I fell asleep.

At this time I did not know Torben had stayed by my side through the night. He watched as the nurses repeatedly drew my blood, and was visited minutes later by the doctor who kept shaking his head, looking at my poor platelet numbers. The possibility of my death was such that a social worker visited with Torben to prepare him for the likelihood.

I next remember Joseph standing quietly by my head. He held a notebook for me. I wrote "Was I really in atrial-ventricular fibrillation?" (Don't know why I wrote "atrial-ventricular," and think I remember only being in atrial fib....But that is beside the point). Torben took one look at the long word I scrawled sloppily across the paper. He admitted to me later that at that moment he thought I was severely brain damaged, thinking I had simply "scribbled the alphabet" in cursive. The nurse took one look at it and said, "That says atrial-ventricular fibrillation. Yes, I believe you were.

In the series of blurs around the room, I saw our friends. Some were crying. Some were hugging Torben. I found it funny at the moment Torben was hugging his buddy, Chris. I wrote on the paper Joseph held for me, "Ha Ha Torben and Chris are hugging." I was still not getting how serious this all was. A couple we had been friends with for a few years were dressed rather nicely. They said they had to go to a funeral. It was close to being mine, I guess.

My next memory is of Tuesday morning, and being in the dark, unable to move my arms. I couldn't figure out why they were tied down at the wrists. It was a horrible feeling. I struggled for a while before I finally opened my eyes and saw I was still in the same room. But it was so quiet now. The clock in front of me above the door read 8:00. I figured it was morning. I kept closing my eyes and opening them. Each time I looked at the clock it said 8:00! It did not budge! "Was it broken?" I wondered. My throat hurt, and I could tell the sleeping drugs were slowly wearing off. Things weren't a dreamy haze, but a solid plop into lucidity. The tube in my throat was now really starting to bug me.

Finally, after what seemed to be an eternity, I fell asleep, at what I still believed to be 8:00. I awoke when the nurses came in at 9:00. They were checking to see if I was ready to have the tube removed. Once I responded in the affirmative, a researcher from the University asked for permission to include me in a study regarding progress made by people taken off respiratory support, based on how well they breathed on their own while the tube was still in, but not connected to the oxygen. "Of course," I wrote and signed the consent form. He seemed elated I was so quick to understand and sign up, and left the room.

The nurses came back and got me ready. They had me take a deep breath in, and then exhale as they pulled the tube out. It hurt *so* much at the time; and I still felt the irritation deep down days later. But boy was it nice not to have it in there.

133

Most of that day I was energized, and even giddy with happiness to be where I was. In retrospect, it must have been the drugs. Visitors came and went, and I laughed and talked all day. My good friend Kathy came. Even little Kirsten was able to come in. I don't recall she took much interest in me though.

Unfortunately, I paid for all the gabbing and laughing the next day. As I moved out of the ICU, I felt the effects and was exhausted and had a very sore throat. I still had a urethral catheter that seemed to kink. It was adjusted by a male nurse. In that position, I tried to think of something clever and witty to say, but couldn't, assuming he had heard it all. My arms were ridiculously swollen, and my left arm, the one with the IVs, was dark red-purple.

My next room was not so fun. I had a roommate who must have thought I enjoyed listening to her talk on the phone. I was really crabby one night when the talking and laughing between a new patient and a nurse went on for hours and never seemed to stop. I remember texting one of my sisters, asking "Did I actually die and go to hell? This is awful!" Yet, all in all I didn't complain too much. The next morning two more friends came bearing a gift, a goofy stuffed yak with a cute tuft of hair on the top of his head. I won't ever part with it.

It wasn't until a few days later that I learned I had received 42 vials of antivenin, half of which came from Missouri, where timber rattlers are a bit more common. The arm they had used to infuse it, the left, had now turned almost black, and had developed a clot in the vein that permanently blocked it. I was a bit anemic, my white cell and platelet counts were low, and my clotting tests were still a bit slow. But they had all been improving at each draw, so I was okayed to go home by the fifth day. I was almost guaranteed to have "serum sickness" a reaction to the antivenin. I did.

By the time of my discharge, my three sisters and mom all converged from Oregon, Georgia, and Minnesota. They picked me up at the hospital and took me out to lunch my first day out. It ended up being a fantastic visit interspersed with hysterical laughter and a bit of crying.

The crying was mostly from me. See, this is where my life as a cliché comes in. After almost dying, at a period in my life when I had taken on too many responsibilities and needed to cut back, I knew I wanted to spend more time with my kids and husband. Animals so often took priority over snuggling on the couch with Kirsten, seeing one of Joseph's choir concerts, making a decent meal for them, or going out on a date with Torben more than semi-annually. I also felt sad I couldn't visit the rest of my family as often as I would have liked.

Those movies about people having near-death experiences eventually quitting their jobs, or cutting back to "do the important things in life," aren't so silly to me anymore. In a very real way I had to do the same. So I am now one of those "Ooh-I've-had-a-life-changing-experience-and-want-to-spend-more-time-with-my-family" people. A cliché. I even dyed my hair pitch black for no apparent reason. What the heck?

I had to disappoint some shelters, and the people there whom I adore, knowing it was going to be very hard for them to find a new vet willing to do shelter work. It was very sad for me. It helped to have my trio of sisters and mom reminding me that it would all work out.

This isn't to say I didn't think long and hard about the amount of time Witty Kitties takes from me. After all, it isn't a paying job, like the others. But unlike the others, it is so much a part of my life that I don't even know where my personal pets or responsibilities end and the shelter begins. Also, so many terrific people have already taken over an amazing number of responsibilities, not to mention the fact that they kept everything going while I was sick. Fortunately, thanks to them, I now clean only a few times a week, and pretty much focus on the medical stuff, doing dentals, blood work, and spays or neuters. I now can be happily oblivious to the phone calls, volunteer organizing, fixing broken "stuff," picking up a new litter supply.

Yes, I gave it a try. I only hoped financially we could work this out. I really did, as I actually liked being able to do chores around here without being in a total rush, being home an extra day of the week, cooking a meal on those nights, not being so tired.

The other of the two quotes I mentioned much earlier? I'm embarrassed to say, I don't know who

Katherine Mansfield is, but only that she said this: "Regret is an appalling waste of energy. You can't build on it; it's only good for wallowing in." Sometimes I'll substitute "Guilt" for the word "Regret," but both suit me just fine. These days, as happily as possible, I go about my days in my new life, cutting back, remembering to pay more attention to the most important things and people, and not getting too unnerved by the smaller paycheck. Hopefully.

Speaking of money, I love asking people if they can guess the total cost of this whole adventure. The cost of the antivenin alone could buy a pretty nice house around here. Of course, since Torben's job provides us with the awesome insurance that is pretty much covering most of it, I am not going to encourage *him* to cut back on *his* work at the post office. Sorry, Sweetie, only one major life change at a time....

Total cost = $245,000.00

If You Build It, They Won't Come

I just had my ass kicked by a 4 ½ foot tall baby emu. Don't let the term "baby" fool you. The legs on those things will kick your nose into your face if you let them. It is snowing and cold at the moment. I am tired. Once again, upon reflection, I am amazed at how much time I put into fruitless ventures. Of course, once again, I know I won't change my behavior one iota.

I sit at the computer desk in our dining/family room, sipping a beer, and shivering a bit because I have yet to change out of my wet clothes. I am typing furiously and truly wish my desire to describe what just happened wasn't stronger than my desire to get myself cleaned up, dry, and warm.

In the last two weeks, I have spent about $2,000 on two structures meant to house and shelter animals who have brains the size of the period at the end of this sentence. Okay, their brains are actually a bit larger than a dot, but not by much.

From where I sit, I can see into our back yard and the area beyond. Dusk is finally setting in and our first big snow, with those big fluffy flakes, is coming down hard. The structures are still visible. One is nothing more than a slanted roof with a single wall on the west and north side. I see the glow of the 250 watt heat lamp I had secured into it. I can almost make out some of the feeders suspended from the many branches I had installed as roosts beneath the roof. The only thing missing are the guinea fowl.

I very purposefully built the structure directly under the tree the guineas roost in every night. I had even cut branches of the same diameter as the ones they favor and had installed them close to the feeders. The feeders are loaded with seeds that I know they love because I've seen them on the deck, emptying birdfeeders of the exact same seed. Another feeder is filled with scratch grains, and another with crumbled poultry feed. I see the guineas about 10 feet above the shelter, sitting in the tree. So far, they are not fooled. For now, I have to accept their rejection and hope they will someday use it.

My consolation is the fact that the guinea structure cost only a few hundred dollars, much less than the other structure, a shed actually. It was built by a friend, but I did the finishing touches. The 12 x 10 foot shed has three walls, a slanted roof, and is at the bottom of the hill in our pasture, close to where the emus built their last few nests. The intention was that the male and baby emus would use it once the weather got colder. Unfortunately, by the time I decided to have the thing built, the daddy emu, Schoonie, had decided he was no longer going to rear his babies. Up until then, he had protected them from everyone and everything, including the momma emu, Flynnie, who still chased and tried to stomp them.

The situation now is that Schoonie and Flynnie are once again an item, scoping out the land for their next nest. Momma still chases her babies but daddy just stands by. This is hard to watch, especially when she chases the smaller one who has balance issues.

Less than a week ago we'd had our first really cold night. It was clear the next morning that the babies were shivering, especially the small one. (Note: I refuse to name them until fully grown. If you name them, they will die. This is one of my superstitions born of experience.) Their backs were covered in frost. It was obvious they had sat fully exposed outside, *not* inside an existing shed with the horse, llamas, and pig. It was then that I decided to have the new shed built, and was thrilled to have it completed in just a few days. The finishing touch would be heavy cattle gates I would mount to the front of the structure.

Yesterday I went to the local farm supply store all grubby in my torn jeans (black leggings underneath), torn sweatshirt, boots, and canvas jacket with blood on the sleeve (don't worry, it was my blood). I like going to the farm store like this because I feel like I won't be viewed as a poser. "Hey, she is tough. She farms," I picture the employees saying. "She knows what she's looking for so I won't bother her." Sometimes it's amazing how much energy I put into not being interrupted by people and what a relief it is when my tactics actually work.

I bought two 6 foot long, and two 8 foot long cattle gates made of 1 ¾ inch metal tubes. After paying the few hundred dollars for the gates, I drove my van to the loading area to meet the person who would assist me.

I own a minivan and had put all the seats down. I knew from experience the gates would fit. I was feeling pretty cool until I saw the guy who was going to load them. I had spoken with him on previous trips to this store. He appeared to be in his 60s. He complained in a smoker's rasp about how he never had help and was the only employee who answered calls for load-outs. He always managed to bring up the fact that he didn't get paid what he deserved and that he shouldn't expect much because of the ethnicity of store's owner. He also managed to work at least one double entendre into any conversations we had. Today I just offered the occasional "yep" once in a while and tried tuning him out.

Once loaded, I drove home, collected my power drill, hammer, etc., and dragged the heavy gates down to the new shed, happy I had picked green ones. "It is a shame this isn't the shed at the top of the hill everyone sees when they drive by," I thought. (The one people could see from the road was built by yours truly, without a plan or knowledge of how to build a shed. I just "Jenni-rigged" it all together, hoping it would still be standing after a year.)

After I hauled the gates and tools down the hill, I measured and drilled holes into the 6 x 6 inch posts for the huge screw-in gate anchors, struggled mightily to actually get the anchors in, then again struggled to lift and secure the gates. When finished, I stood back and admired the work. It looked great! My plan was to keep these gates open, then make another wall with the remaining two 6 foot gates.   This would provide both a shelter and an outside area for the emus during the winter.

Finally, I got to spend a fruitless hour or so trying to lure the baby emus into the shed. What usually works is food; but that was stupid. Where there is food there will also be the llamas, the adult emus, the donkey, etc. I bagged the idea and put some straw into the shed and called it quits, hoping the babies would somehow figure out this was a better place to nestle in for the night than the open pasture.

During chores the next morning, I performed my daily ritual: Pellets for horse, llamas, and donkey into separate feeders, then toss out food for ducks, geese, and pig. Next I intended to feed the adult emus, who usually eat near the mammals. Not today. This morning they were in the baby emus' usual spot at the corner of our big shed, where the fence to the pasture is attached. Their spot is also near the entrance to a long pen that ran along the length of the building (Initially built to house a silver fox, and later some dogs. It now stood empty).

I refused to feed the adults emus until they left that spot. In the meantime the babies were wandering aimlessly, looking for food. When the llamas came along after eating their rations, the adult emus finally moved to their usual place. But now the llamas were in the baby emu feeding spot! The babies were getting a bit crazy, pacing further out in the pasture.

I called the llamas, "Lorennnnnzo! Sparrrrrrkles!" and coaxed them back to their feed buckets which I had filled with a second ration of pellets. Of course by now Willow (the horse) and Pasado (the naughty, wild donkey) had finished theirs and had to be given seconds as well. I just wanted them to stay put! Finally, the adult emus began eating food in their regular spot. But the babies were still lost. They had moved closer to Pasado. When I started shooing them along, Pasado, who will not let you touch him without force, thought I was chasing *him*. He got all stupid and took it out on the baby emus by snapping at them. I kept walking with my face turned away from the donkey, hoping he would think "Hey, she ain't lookin' at me. I should calm the heck down." That eventually worked.

Several minutes later, the baby emus were near their feeding station. They still did not want to eat in their normal spot because of an extra fence panel I had put up the night before; the panel effectively made a space that was walled off on three sides. It is not in an emu's nature to let itself be cornered, so they hesitated when they got close. Frustrated, I walked far away while I watched. Eventually one baby, and then the other, went into the corner to eat. As they ate, I gave them a wide berth before coming back and pushing a fourth panel into place so they were enclosed.

At this point, the baby emus could stand there and eat, walk into the old fox pen, or get all frantic and start banging against the fence panels to escape. After much frantic banging around, they went into the pen.

Relieved, I closed the door and did a dance. I was done with step one. I gave them water and some food and decided to wait until tomorrow to recruit someone to help me move them to the new shed at the bottom of the hill.

So I thought.

As the day went on (a Saturday) it got really cloudy; the snow that was predicted started coming down. I was impatient and kept thinking about how the baby emus were just standing out in the open even while in the fox pen. They were getting covered in snowflakes and ignoring the straw I had put up against the shed for them. I bit the bullet, went into the pen, and chased down the bigger of the two. The bird ran and threw itself against the fence, the way they do when feeling threatened. I finally jumped on it, only to have it fall and roll over onto its back. That is when the powerful, skull-crushing kicks began. I forced the feet beneath my arms and turned it around. It was too strong. There was no way I was holding its legs AND getting it out of the pen AND moving it down the hill. I left to think this over some more.

After much mulling, I returned with an old bed sheet. This time I got the smaller of the two. This one slipped and fell due to its balance issue, making it easy to catch. It too kicked like a terror until I wrapped the sheet around its legs and body. I managed to open the gate, go through it, and latch it again while holding the struggling beast against me. I made it down the hill, wondering why I was doing this; I didn't anticipate being able to transfer the bigger, much stronger one. I went into the new little shed, closed the gate behind me, then fell onto the ground with the baby emu still in my arms. It quickly struggled out of the sheet, rammed into the gate, then pushed itself sideways through the 12 inch space between the bars. While this was happening I just stood there in disbelief, capable of stopping it, but too dumbfounded to move my feet. I watched as it popped out onto the other side of the gate, got up, and staggered away.

Now I had a stressed baby emu I needed to catch. I worried about the fact that emus can be stressed to the point of death. The stress the babies would feel at being on the opposite sides of the fence from each other was also a concern. They were both pacing now, trying to be with each other. After two runs up the hill, out of breath, and down, then up again, I finally got close enough to the emu. Feeling guilty at having to be so rough after all it had been through, I fell onto it, grabbed it from behind, and let it kick all it wanted. Somehow I then got it up the hill and back into the old fox pen; the baby emus were reunited. Unfortunately, they had planted themselves at the fully exposed southern end of the enclosure.

I needed a new plan.

I thought some more, then realized I could take advantage of the alterations I had made to the pen on a previous occasion. Although I originally built this pen for a fox, it was pretty much a super long dog run. When we took in six dogs as a favor to a local shelter, I had to make some alterations. The dogs couldn't all be together, so I put up a short gated that separated the long enclosure into two equal halves. I then divided the north half into two halves. Even divided in this way, the quarter portions were much larger than a typical dog run.

The emus were still standing at the exposed south end; I decided I needed to close off that half of the pen. Before doing this, I made the north half as attractive as possible for two cold, young emus. I put a tarp over a portion of it, a piece of plywood to block the chilly north wind, much straw on the ground, a pail for water, a pile of food, and heat lamp with protective screen. Once done, I left for a while, assuming the emus would be curious and discover the food, wander in, feel how warm it was, then fall in love with it and stay put. I could then simply shut the gate in the middle of the enclosure so they wouldn't wander into the exposed area during the night.

An hour later when it started getting dark, I returned feeling hopeful, but they were still out in the open on the south end, getting covered with snow. I then went in and walked towards them, essentially scaring them into getting away from me while allowing them to run past me to the north, warmer end of the enclosure. I then kicked and jiggled the gate that separated the two halves of the pen out of the icy ground and closed it. About a third of their new smaller area was covered and heated. I wanted to think they would suddenly realize how much warmer it felt, but they were running in circles and bouncing off each other; they seemed fearful I was about to kill them or something. The smaller one actually fell backwards and onto its side, kicking frantically before finally getting itself up.

My problem now was the fact that the emus were in their little frenzy, and they separated me from the pen's exit at the north end. Fearing I would cause them to go into convulsions if I tried to walk past them to get out, I decided it would be kinder if I climbed over the fence, which I will remind you is 6 feet high. Contemplating the fence, and the fact that I had big boots on, and that the top of the fence leaned inwards a bit, I stood there hoping the babies would suddenly calm down, or better yet, would sit under the lamp and fall asleep. Instead, they stood at the gate running their beaks back and forth against the chain-link.

By now it was completely dark except for a distant yard light. I was getting cold, so up and over the fence I went. As usual, when climbing over a high fence I couldn't help but worry that part of my clothing would get stuck on it, so when I dropped down I do so only partially and the rest of me hangs there. It reminds me of my favorite scene from *Napolean Dynamite*, the one where Napolean, who is running from his uncle, climbs over the fence and falls clumsily over the other side. For me, this time, I was fine. I dropped as softly as a 52 year old woman in big Muck books can drop from a 6 foot fence. No one was watching. That was good.

So, I sit here hoping the guinea fowl and emu sheds are not all in vain. My new larger shed is not working for the baby emus for now. They are at least enclosed in a smaller area where they have the option of staying warm and dry. I know that when I head out to do chores in the Witty Kitties shelter building beyond the pasture and pens, I must stop myself from peeking in the direction of the baby emus. What would I do if they are again not under the lamp but out in the exposed portion of their small pen? It is late, and there are other animals to care for. I am still wet and my beer is finished. Tomorrow morning will, I suppose, reveal who really has a brain the size of a ".".

Reconstructionist Theory: Maggie and Morgan, Two Case Histories

It's a funny thing — several years ago, during a couple week time period, I worked on two cases that were very similar, but had totally different outcomes. I'm still not sure I understand why.

Maggie was a Basenji mix, about a year old, who suffered a close-range shotgun injury a month prior. She was a stray dog, very timid, and difficult to catch. Thanks to good Samaritans, she was finally lassoed and brought in to a local shelter. The poor dog was missing literally inches of muscle from over her shoulders. The "spinous process" of one of her vertebrae was gone; the splinters of bone were just scattered around, as were splinters from the edge of one of her scapulae. What they were scattered about in was a combination of dead tissue, serum, purulent discharge ("pus"), and maggots (not just the tiny ones, either). It was a hot summer. I wasn't too surprised.

In cases like this, where a wound has festered so long that remaining tissue is dead or contaminated, the first goal, assuming the animal is strong enough for anesthesia, is to debride (clean) it. This procedure involves: 1) an anesthetized dog; 2) quality latex gloves that won't tear willy-nilly, leaving you with gore under your fingernails you don't realize is there until well into the procedure; 3) tissue scissors, scalpel, gauze, and lots of saline for flushing the area. In retrospect, an entire face shield would have been nice but I didn't want the folks at the Iowa City shelter, where she stayed initially, to think I had gone soft on them.

Cleaning **Maggie's** wound is for sure in my top five grossest things I've ever had to do. I would love to share the details of the different species of fly larvae and how they were each stationed in different ways in the tissue, but that would just be gratuitous. Wouldn't it? You sure? Never mind. Here goes.

The most populous of **Maggie's** maggots were the tiny ones most of us who pay attention to such things recognize as housefly larvae. They and the eggs from which they hatch, are relatively tiny and tend to occur in clumps here and there on the wound. I can't even tell you how many wounds and sores I've seen that have had maggots such as these. The animals never seem to notice; and the larvae provide a bit of assistance by feeding on the necrotic (dead) tissue.

Blow fly larvae are much bigger than the wimpy housefly larvae and have disgusting little barb rings around their bodies. I found them in what looked like a pod colony from an alien movie; all of the fat little grubs sunken nicely into the little chambers they had made themselves pretty much by eating their way down into the tissue.

Finally, the bluebottle flies were dispersed throughout the area, moving and squirming within the soup of gore that used to be the dog's poor back.

Poor Maggie had no idea she was hosting a pool party up there, carrying it along wherever she went, not really paying it much attention actually.

My second patient, a cat named **Morgan**, was also a stray; he was finally captured by a kindhearted person after much difficulty. **Morgan** was missing 75% of the skin from the circumference of his neck; a band over 2 inches wide wound around from below one ear, down, and over to the other. The wound was weeks old. It was so chronic that once I removed all the dried pus, dead skin, dirt, and plant material that had decided to tag along for the ride, I saw that the skin at portions of the wound edges had a smooth, healed connection with the exposed tissue. His body was trying hard to heal itself; the skin had moved inward towards the wound as far as it could go in some portions.

It was obvious the wound had been much larger previously, as there was a subtle tension at the edges where the skin and wound line appeared "healed" to each other (no other way of explaining it). If it hadn't been for the fact that the poor cat was losing a large amount of fluids and protein from the wound site I would have thought he was doing a fairly good job of healing without my help. So, just as with **Maggie,** I flushed and cut and cleaned and then lectured the cat (under anesthesia of course) that he had to keep healing himself until the wound was small enough for me to close the gap, preferably without a graft.

Maggie, the dog, wouldn't eat her antibiotics, so had to have pricey injections that would hopefully cover what bacteria were living in her wound.

Morgan, the cat, also got the same shot, as he wouldn't consistently take all his meds in his food, and was too wild to be pilled.

A week after **Maggie** arrived I knocked her out again for her second surgery to close the wound up. An absolute rule in closing skin wounds or surgical incisions is that there should be no tension whatsoever on the skin sutures. Deeper layers of tissue have to be closed one after the other until you have apposition that allows the skin sutures or skin staples to sit nicely without pulling. The goal is to have no pulling at the site, which is very uncomfortable for the animal. There were portions of the void I could not pull together without making relief incisions near the wound. (Relief incisions are cuts into the skin a bit away from the wound at the area with the most tension.) The incision can be a simple line which is closed perpendicular to the cut, or a "Z" incision which is then sutured in a way that brings skin closer to the wound without taking too much from its source. You can get really inventive with them. As I recall, I consulted surgery text and found which best suited Maggie's injury. In the end, she had multiple lines all connecting at the same site, or close to it. I felt I had left a minimal amount tension on the skin in a few areas and none in most, but still was really paranoid about the wound opening up again. I held my breath.

Meanwhile, my first attempt at **Morgan**'s neck reconstruction was not as well-planned-out a process. Shortly after sedating him, yet not completely anesthetizing him, I reversed a portion of his sedative once I realized that I needed to do some research. I spent that evening reviewing reconstruction/skin flaps in that same surgery book. The next day I gave it a go. I cut enormous patches of skin from each side of his shoulder/chest area, and swung them around, thus having a nice bunch of skin to cover the defects without tension. The donor sites closed easily (hey, just like the book said they would!). I felt really good about how it went. I had not done such extensive movement of skin and was confident Morgan was going to heal very well. There was not a bit of tension anywhere.

Almost two weeks later I stopped holding my breath. **Maggie's** shoulder injury site was lovely, and almost ready to have the staples and sutures removed. Now that she was medically sound, we could work harder on her socialization and make her a good future pet for some lucky people. Looking at her now, I couldn't imagine the area being as bad as I remembered.

Not so for **Morgan**. Unfortunately his neck area became infected, thus preventing healing, and all of his incisions opened up after a week, making his situation much worse that it had been before.

I had a dilemma. Half measures weren't going to take care of **Morgan's** injury. If I wanted to have a happy ending I would need to culture the area and send it to a lab to determine which antibiotics would take care of the problem. Then I'd need to figure out how to get the antibiotics into him without traumatizing him on a daily basis, as he was only now letting me clean his cage and feed him without smacking my hand with his paw. I really wanted to be able to call this a success, and thought about how darned proud I'd be of myself.

Damn. I said that word. "Proud." Pride is a problem.

Whenever I find myself thinking like this, I get really hard to live with. I spent all day sulking, not necessarily about the fact that I may not be able to heal this cat, but because I wasn't sure of my motivation at this stage. The thought of relieving his discomfort after so long, and maybe even having him appreciate being cared for, is all I wanted when I first met **Morgan,** as well as **Maggie**. But now I didn't know if one more attempt was in his best interest. After the flap surgery, he was in a lot of pain. My gut was telling me he now had much less than a 50:50 chance of survival considering his reluctance to take medication. The best antibiotics would probably not be available in convenient injections, or be tasty enough to hide in his food. Compounding pharmacies were not the norm back then. So, all this being true, my going ahead with continuing to treat him would be more for me than for him.

After giving **Morgan** his treat of canned food, which had become an expected pleasure for him in the evenings, and with euthanasia in the back of my mind, I snuck my hand into his cage and injected a heavy sedative in his muscle. After a hiss and a smack, he went back to eating. I watched him as he simultaneously ate and slowly went to sleep, his head going down, down, down. This is how I prefer to euthanize any animal, allow it to just eat until his/her head falls right into its food. At that point I give the actual euthanasia solution injection which puts the animal deeper under, until the breathing and then the heart stops.

Sidebar: Whenever I hear about botched executions I wonder why prisons don't use this technique. I am not stating I am for capital punishment,; but IF it is done, just give people a heavy sedative, let them eat their favorite meal, then give the fatal injection. I am not trivializing the process, just trying to show that it would sure make more sense. I once stopped on the side of the highway while on my way to work one morning, on hold with NPR's "On Point" show one morning. The topic was botched executions. After sitting on hold for a good 20 minutes I was suddenly talking to Tom Ashbrook, and being asked what I had to say. I went on to tell him I was a veterinarian and how I felt we vets had this euthanasia thing down. Why couldn't our method be done with humans? (Again, I am NOT stating my opinion of capital punishment.) Tom actually agreed with me! His guest brought up euthanizing his own dog and that I had a point. After signing off, I went happily on my way, thinking I had done a huge service to the world and that my idea would make a difference because so many people listened to NPR my idea would make a difference. That was over 10 years ago.

Back to sad **Morgan**.

Once I was certain Morgan was completely asleep I took a closer look at his wound, removing the discharge and dead tissue. What I saw left me confident the next step was the right choice. I gave Morgan the euthanasia injection and let him go.

Not really sure why I ended up crying afterwards. It just have been because Morgan had suffered so long, and didn't have a chance to live a normal life. Or it was because I had failed him. Or it could have been because I was actually in a mindset earlier that put my pride ahead of his welfare. After a heck of a lot of work, my efforts were in vain. Regardless, after making sure he was gone, and covering him up with his blankets so I could remove him in the morning, I decided to walk outside. I took a deep breath, and went to the back of the Witty Kitties shelter where **Maggie** was being kept in a long dog run on my property. I sat near her a while, and smiled. Her wound was now a scar and she was ready for the next stage in her life, getting a new forever home. Her shy brown eyes never told me she was particularly pleased with my presence; they had a soft gentleness still mixed with a bit of fear I think. She was a tough nut to crack.

During this time one of our most loyal Witty Kittties' volunteers had been going back to Maggie's run to talk to her, and several weeks later took her home for good. Lora is a retired school teacher; she and her husband favor taking in hard dog cases and do very well at it. **Maggie Maggot Dog** is still around, and coincidently lives only a few miles away. I periodically see her on visits to the home. She still will not allow me to approach her. I am fine with that. She is comfortable and has the home any dog could love.

Rearranging Memories (Close Encounters – The Deer Story)

It's funny how my memory of an incident can change each time I think about it. I am sure no one truly remembers things exactly as they happen considering all the variables that affect how we visualize and interpret things. As these variables can change, so can our assessment or opinion of any given event.

Typically, if I do something dumb or embarrassing, I can't stand it. I want it to disappear. I hope no one witnessed it. Don't want to be seen as dumb as I feel. Yet at the same time, I'll replay the incident over and over in my mind, hoping maybe it wasn't as bad as I initially thought, picking out a different detail each time, thus driving myself crazy. Once I've overanalyzed it and recalled the details, I try altering it a bit, in hopes that I can train my memory to remember it as being not quite as bad as it really was, helping me get over it and (hopefully) forget it entirely, thus preserving my self-esteem.

That never works. Memories of my being dumb always set in like stone.

But years ago I had an incident which, when I think about it, gets more and more bizarre every time I think about it. I didn't have the immediate feeling that I had done anything stupid at the time, nor did I immediately afterwards, so had no plan to obsess over it. I had an interesting event occur and I liked telling people about it. However, with each telling of the story, I realized more and more just how foolish I had been. After telling the story many times over, I knew I had indeed done a dumb thing; the details therefore would not go away. But I do find myself going over and over it even today, just to prove to myself how bloody lucky I was.

The incident happened early in November. My son Joseph was in a high school musical and did not have a car. I had been making two round trips to his school, three days a week, for practice. I would take him around 5:00 p.m. or so and pick him up around 9:00. It was always really dark for the later drive. And, being early November, it was also deer hunting season and rutting season for the white-tailed deer which are abundant in our area. The ten mile drive started out on a gravel back road which then turned into a paved county road. Because deer are always an issue in this area and because they were especially active this time of year I was used to keeping my eyes peeled for any running across the road.

This year the deer population was especially high, so on this particular night, when I saw a large deer standing in the middle of the road at the top of a hill ahead of me, I wasn't too shocked. I saw it silhouetted first, as an oncoming car went right past it. Oddly, the deer just stood there. As I got closer, I noticed a large antler laying in my lane. The deer, standing on the middle line of the road, had only one on his head. I drove within a few yards of it, staying in my lane. He just stood staring at me. Assuming he was temporarily stunned after being bumped by a car (which obviously explained his broken antler), I figured he just needed to be scared off. I honked my horn and flicked my lights a few times. He just stood there.

So I pulled onto the shoulder, stopped my engine, but kept my headlights on for some indirect light. When I got out of the van I noticed the silence and stillness of the night, disturbed only by the buck's heavy breathing. I just stood there dumbfounded, as he turned his head towards me and looked right at me. I waved my arms and yelled at him to scare him off the road, but he still stood there staring at me. Assuming my walking towards him would scare him, I did just that. Would you believe he still stood just there?

I kept walking until I was next to him. At this point I had forgotten my goal to get him off the road, and fell into a spell over what an amazing beast he was! This is where I get really stupid. I started rubbing his head and neck, like I would a horse. I was just so struck by how muscular and dense he was. I couldn't believe how HUGE he was! And I was petting him!

For those of you who are not familiar with what could have happened to me, I will explain. I was standing there with my guard down; I was petting a male deer during rutting season like I would a baby unicorn on a fluffy cloud. An angry buck can stand up on his back legs and pretty much drive his hooves into your face or gut, not to mention impale you with those antlers as easily as you put a stick into a marshmallow before roasting it. I was not using common sense.

From the top of the hill I saw another car coming about a mile away in the opposite lane. Quickly I tried pushing the buck to the shoulder of the road. He wouldn't go. I got behind him and slapped his rump, hoping deer don't kick like horses do. He still stood there in a daze. His breathing got no more or less labored. Then I managed to figure out how to be even dumber and I went **in front** of him and started pulling on his one antler! He still just stayed put. As the oncoming car got closer, I again got behind him and started hitting his rear really hard and screaming at him. This seemed to startle him enough to take a couple of steps to the side of the road. There we stood, side-by-side, and watched the car pass by without even a tap to the brakes.

"Hey, look honey! There is a woman with her pet deer standing by the road." ZOOM!

Suddenly I seemed to be out of whatever daze I'd been in and my veterinarian brain started thinking about what more this poor deer may need. Is he more damaged than I thought? Did he need steroids? What type of harm occurred elsewhere? How is his chest? Could I somehow get an X-ray? How do I get him in my van? We have had goats, llamas, and adult emus in the minivan. Why not an enormous buck?

I thought Torben could come and help me get him in his pickup. I even went so far as to dial our home number, then hung up when it rang, finally realizing how ridiculous this was. The thought of a deer tolerating being put into a vehicle was ludicrous.

Needless to say, I had momentarily forgotten about picking up my Joseph. Sadly, it wasn't the first time my mom brain was completely shut down in the face of an injured animal, and wouldn't be the last. So I stood there and kept stroking his side. No blood from his nose or mouth. His breathing was not as labored now. I tried to push him into the ditch. He took a few steps, and looked around. I was happy with that and decided he was coming around. I walked over to the antler on the road and picked it up, knowing I had to have proof of the whole event.

I picked up Joseph, of course going right into my story for the first of many times, before asking, "How was practice my good son?" Driving back on the same road, I saw that the deer was no longer at the spot where I had left him. I hoped he had finally come to his senses and been able to navigate to wherever he needed to be. On that note, I've come to my senses and realize my luck in not having been gored by an antler of an injured male deer during the most stressful time of year.

Despite exposing my stupidity, I still am fascinated by that night and can remember it as though it happened yesterday.

The Interstate Boar:
A Real Road Hog

Just when you think nothing else could happen in your life to make you feel like you have gone over to a surreal world you discover you weren't even close.... until the next event. THEN you feel like, "Okay, now I've seen it all." These events can be fun, or utterly horrible. This story and the next are one of each.

Several summers ago, I had an experience that could have gone either way. On a hot summer day while at work at the Iowa City Animal Care Center, I was finishing up on another long day of surgery, when I overheard something about a pig running loose somewhere. It didn't strike me as strange. Unfortunately, I've seen half a dozen little farm pigs that have fallen off trucks, or just slipped away from a truck while stopped. They were usually the cute little pink ones, all sad and scraped up, but at least they were out of the factory food chain.

I went about my work, when several minutes later I heard that the animal control officer needed the Shelter Director to assist. Huh, odd. But I kept to my line of thought, trying to concentrate on surgery. A short time later a staff person told me I was needed to help get in getting a really large pig sedated and off the busy road he was near. At the moment it didn't occur to me just HOW BIG the pig would be, and HOW BUSY the road would be. I grabbed my stuff, feeling excited fabout doing something out of the ordinary.

While driving to the location I was told by cell phone the pig was several hundred pounds. Wow! I then got instructions on how to find it. I was to go west on Interstate 80 off Hwy 1 exit ....get into left lane......left lane?.......Okay. Then slowly, really slowly, drive into the median and continue driving between the huge temporary concrete walls. This part of the freeway was a construction site, full of heavy equipment, cones and barriers, huge piles of dirt.......and a pig. I was warned about how bumpy it would be, and felt, while driving between opposing directions of traffic, that this was going to be special.

I finally saw a cop car, an animal control vehicle, and some really big earth moving equipment all bunched together forming a corral of sorts. At the center was my pig.

Mind you, we are talking about 800 lbs of big boar!

Apparently, mysteriously, this pig got loose from God-knows-where, and had made his way onto the interstate just north of Iowa City. He had stopped traffic and caused several folks to call 911. Fortunately, the road construction crew, out of benevolence towards the pig and/or the poor soul who may actually hit the pig, got it into the median and down into the work area. The area stretched almost a mile, and was bordered by those concrete walls. It was a fortunate place to be if you're a pig lost amongst heavy traffic.

By the time I arrived the poor thing had been running in the hot sun for quite a long time. Not good for a pig. One of the construction crew drove the water truck over to spray him with water. When I got there he was on his side, exhausted, and panting. I tried making a bit of shade over him, then got to work.

What did I do? Well, in my shorts and Keen sandals (Yes, some shelter vets get to dress down. At least this one does.), I got to jump into the slimy, muddy, and somewhat poopy stuff surrounding the pig and check him out. Then I pulled up an amount of sedative I thought was enough for just 200 pounds I wasn't sure how much stress he was under, so felt I needed to be careful and not overdose the poor guy. After nothing happened, I gave him another 200 pounds worth, then another.

I had used almost every drop of sedation I had, not surprising since this pig represented days' worth of dogs and cats! I did finally get him to sleep. In case you wonder **why** he needed to sleep, I'll tell you. It was because there was no way to get a vehicle and/or a trailer with a ramp that a hog could walk up into the area we were in. There would be no walking for this guy. We had to move him ourselves. Dead weight.

Great.

With Iowa City being fairly large and progressive, and with the police officers and very kind county construction guys all involved, you'd think, "Oh, the city will come and hoist him up, and carry him off to some wonderful fairy tale farm far away".

No way. With no options out there, at times like this I call my husband, Torben.

It was a Friday, Torben's day off at the time. Figuring I'd ruin it, I called him.

"Hey, can we transport a billion pound pig to our place? Yes, in our little pickup truck."

Now how many women have made a request like that to their husband, expecting a positive response at the drop of a hat?

Being the animal lover he is, and the optimistic say-yes-to-anything-and-not-worry-about-details-til-later type guy, he hopped in his pickup headed on down to meet me from about 20 minutes away.

I then wondered where we would take this pig, so called one of our best friends, Chris, and left a message with him.

"Will you take a billion pound boar off my hands? He has no where to go. Doubt we'll find the owner." So far, no pig I've dealt with after falling off a truck has ever been claimed.

A city truck was able to get into the area to hoist the pig high enough for us to get it level with the back of our not-so-huge pickup truck, a Ford Ranger with a topper. The cops, the city guy, the construction guys were all saying "There is NO way we are going to get this huge thing into that little truck!"

This challenge was enough to give Torben the energy to crawl into the back of the pickup (not easy for a 6' 2", 230 pound, guy) and pull the pig's back (or was it front?) legs, as the few of us willing to get any smellier and muddier pushed. Once in, the boar was the length of the bed of the truck, a bit snug. We closed the tailgate, and flap of the topper, and then....he was Torben's and my problem.

If you had been on the freeway, whizzing by, there is no way you would have known this scenario was going on. The construction area was lower than the road and protected by the concrete walls. Of course, if I stood up on the edge, I had a great view of the cars and trucks cruising on by at a safe 70 mph. It was when I did this that I thought, "Huh, who would have guessed?" It was indeed surreal.

Since the truck's tailgate had been known to pop open periodically, I prayed and prayed the pig wouldn't wake up during the trip and kick right out, only to end up on the freeway again. I had hoped Torben would choose the local highway, less traffic, slower, but he wanted to get home as quickly as possible, so from I-80, he hopped onto I-380. I followed him, hoping and sweating and praying there would not be a headline in the papers the next morning: "Hog survives first episode on freeway, but becomes bacon on second." I also fantasized about the vehicles that would hit him, and the safety of those inside. Who would have the liability and responsibility? This sadly is not the first time I've felt I was in way over my head (remember B-Bear?).

On the road I got a call from our friend Chris, who was willing to take in this poor pig. He had a soft spot for pigs, and was still sad about one he had lost not long ago. He and his wife lived only two miles from us which was helpful.

At this point Torben still thought the pig was going to stay at our home. Where? Beats me! (Again, think B-Bear.) I kept trying to ring Torben on his cell. Kept redialing and redialing...He never answered, which really ticked me off. What if the truck's topper flap had opened? What could he be doing that was more important than making sure we didn't kill the pig and any people who may hit him? I took very little comfort in knowing I would be the first to hit him, thinking maybe I could minimize the damage.

It wasn't until we got into our driveway thatI got Torben's attention.

I shouted from my van, "Chris will take him!"

"But why can't we have him?" Torben asked.

"Shut your pie hole and get over to Chris's!" was my reply.

At this point I must mention another complication that added to my stress level. Our 5 year old daughter Kirsten was due to arrive home from school on the bus at 3:55. Someone had to be there for her. On the drive I called my teenage son, Joseph, who was staying with his dad that evening in Iowa City, to see if he could drive home to meet her. I couldn't reach him, so I called his dad to see if it was Okay for him to do so. All this calling while on the freeway went against my rule of "no phone on the freeway."

Despite all my calling, I reached neither Joseph nor his dad.

The bus was due at our driveway any second.

As soon as Torben headed to Chris's, I ran into the basement, smelling to high heaven of hog, showered, and ran out to the mailbox at the exact moment

Kirsten's bus pulled up. I then swept her up and plopped her back into my van.

"Mom, why does it smell so bad in here?!"

"Never mind, we're going to Uncle Chris's house."

No more questions asked.

I'm not sure if they rolled him out, had him walk, or what, but by the time I got to Chris's the pig was in a former horse stall Chris had reinforced with hog panels. He had space, mud, food, and would soon feel like he was on vacation.

So, things quieted down. Kat (Chris's wife) was happy to have yet another animal thanks to us. It happened all the time and had not cost us her friendship, yet. As a matter of fact during a previous summer, a guy brought us a fawn he had found in a ditch. When we told him to take it back to the ditch he couldn't remember exactly where he found the poor thing. It was probably just waiting for its momma and now it would need fostering to survive. We drove up to Chris and Kat's house, saw them sitting on their upstairs deck, enjoying the day, some wine, Kat's birthday... and said "Happy Birthday!" We gave her the fawn and said "Good Luck with that." And left. Okay, it wasn't that callous, but Kat was actually thrilled, having never touched a fawn; Chris was just as much an animal lover as well. They took the job on, and nursed the fawn along to a point where she could go to a rehabber. Before the fawn, we had "gifted" them cats, ferrets, and later, raccoons. Always good sports, they took them on happily. This obviously helped Torben and me immensely, as we had enough of a menagerie.

A few days passed. Chris had named the pig "Melvin Melon Balls" for obvious reasons. Melvin enjoyed his space, lounged about, and consumed whatever the heck he wanted. He was doted on, and loved. As usual, I charged the Shelter for the cost of my drugs, but not my time, the gas Torben used, etc. Recoup cost for my time was something that was usually an afterthought. It seems like the excitement was well worth it.

Then I got a call from the shelter director. "Jen, do you have a bill? An owner was located, and wants the pig back." NO WAY! I couldn't believe it! No one ever claimed a pig that fell off a truck, especially one that ended up being such a hassle. Who wanted to pay for all that? I mean surely the county would expect money for all the down time spent by the construction guys and machines. Who could pay that?!

Well, it ended up the county didn't charge, though the construction crew got their wages. The police didn't charge, as this was all part of the job. So, it was up to me, Chris, and the shelter to put together a bill. I personally didn't know what a "normal vet" would charge, and even called a local clinic for an opinion. I put together a bill, as did Chris and the shelter. It wasn't huge, but good payment. I figured there was no way in heck anyone would pay for this pig.

Well the "anyone" happened to be an extremely large and popular sausage company that had recently purchased the pig. The driver transporting him and others never noticed him missing. How he got out of the vehicle is anyone's guess. But, in the end, Melvin's "Melon Balls" were valuable, and he was picked up quickly and taken to his new home, hopefully for some fun.

So, another animal had come and gone. We managed to throw another bizarre thing into our lives, something to reminisce about over drinks in Kat and Chris's living room some evenings. We've even toasted the adventuresome pig. Here's to you, Melvin Melon Balls!

It's Not Easy Being Green

Or so it may seem. Kermit the Frog lamented his color in this classic song from The Muppet Movie only to discover he is pretty happy after all, and wouldn't change it if he could.

It's a catchy phrase, "It's not easy being green," and many environmentally conscious folks have picked it up from that 70s icon, indicating a responsibility to the earth. This sentiment could also be referred to as "shrinking your carbon footprint," "recycling," "exploring sustainability"....and on and on. I think it's pretty common to want what is best for the planet and we all need to do what we feel we can to protect it. But as indicated earlier it is indeed NOT easy.

I do a bit to help, recycling cans and pop bottles, reusing containers from certain grocery store items. One thing I love is that rarely does any food go wasted here, as we have a variety of mammals, reptiles, and birds who will eat scraps or unwanted leftovers. That part of green living is easy for me. Who wants food going to waste? I've heard composting can be kind of tedious at times; doubt I will ever find out myself since the only things we can't seem to get our "living garbage disposals" to eat is onions.

At times we have taken recycling a step further. If a chicken or duck is killed by a wild raccoon (or even by a certain mastiff who fooled us into thinking she wasn't interested in them the first week we had her) or dies naturally, we make sure someone on the farm gets to eat it. Once you get past the "icky" factor, it is all right. But when a llama passes, or when I've put down a pony, we haven't done the most environmentally sound disposal. I've always had them cremated. They're big. And digging any-size hole is very difficult in our clay soil. Also, eating horse and llama isn't something we are willing to do. That's too "icky" for us, though I know some people might not think so.

It is because I believe cremation isn't good for the environment that I recently purchased two small backhoes attachments for a bobcat. Before you think we have money to burn I must tell you that we don't actually own the machinery to operate the backhoes, just the actual scooper things. My friend and co-worker, Nancy, owns a landscape business. Her business owns a small walk-behind bobcat. I "loaned" her the backhoes so she could use them for her business. In return we agreed that I could call her whenever one of our big animals died. I know that already this fall she used the backhoes to dig a grave for another friend's pony when he passed. Nancy and "The Grave Digger" can usually accommodate a burial within 24 hours. Buying the backhoe was a good investment, and I feel better about the more environmentally sound disposal. Also, Nancy may be able to have fun with The Grave Diggers for other more pleasant uses as well.

But once in a while we have the passing of a large animal that **is** customarily raised for food, and actually had been going that route before it made its way to us. What does one do? I found out what I would do when I acquired, and subsequently lost, the phenomenal creature we called Apples the Pig.

Apples was a small farm piglet we got from the local municipal shelter after she fell off a transport truck onto a highway outside town. This sounds outrageous because it **is** outrageous, but it is not uncommon. I can remember at least half dozen farm-pig-falling-out-of-the-truck incidents in the last ten years. How people can transport pigs in a way that allows them to come tumbling out onto the road is beyond me. Is it just a given that one or two will pop out in transport and be considered a routine loss? I just don't get it. It is not unlike the expected mortality of chickens and turkeys being transported long distances. An acceptable number die due to heat, cold, and stress. It is sad.

At the time she fell, Apples was just a piglet; her little body was covered in road rash and ticks. We happily took her in one May when we still lived in our old farmhouse. The first day I had her, Kirsten had t-ball practice at school. She was only in first grade yet had already learned that her mom was not like all the other moms. She did not blink an eye when I arrived at practice with a little scratched up pig on a harness and leash. Her friends reminded her how lucky she was to have such a "cool mom," but from her reaction, I knew she saw yet one more animal who would take me away from her.

Jennifer Doll

Previous farm pigs we've had (most also had fallen out of trucks) had been adopted and gone on to wonderful lives. After having her for several weeks without inquiries, we decided to keep Apples as our own. She was a lot of fun. She arrived a few weeks before two coyote pups (raised in a gentleman's home) came to us; the three frequently played together, until Apples bit too hard and set the pups running scared. As Apples grew, the number of animals she could hang out with got smaller and smaller due to her size and rough play. The places we could keep her were fewer and fewer as well. She spent most of her time in the main yard that surrounded our house (which was already showing the effects of having livestock rubbing up against it). She even stayed inside our house early on.

Apples was actually pretty dog-like in her behavior and seemed to like following me on my rounds during morning chore time. I have fond memories of taking her through the large animal pasture on the way to the building where the Witty Kitties shelter is housed. At that time, Apples was still too little to live with the big livestock. As I did the chores, she ran and skipped around me happily. This went on every morning, until she was discovered by Pasado the Evil Donkey. Pasado is as mean as he is cute, and he is REALLY cute! He decided one day he needed to start chasing Apples and try to stomp on her. He did this with any new smaller animal that set foot in the pasture, be it a dog, cat, goat, or, as it turns out, pig. His only exception for some reason was possums, which happen to be my favorite of all animals. So, if you were new and small and not a possum, and in his pasture

174

you had to be put in your place. That place was under his foot!

The emus and llamas usually behaved similar to Pasado, but for some reason let Pasado have all the fun when it came to Apples. My favorite image of Apples is her racing at the fastest pace she could go from the top of the hill by the shelter, down through the pasture and up to the gate nearer our house, squealing all the way, after Pasado startled her from behind a tree.

I eventually had to put her on the leash. Pasado is pretty feral and won't get too near me, so he threatened a leashed Apples only from a distance. Unfortunately for me however, if Pasado stomped his feet even far away, Apples would spin around and around me, wrapping me with the leash. I made chores even more difficult since I'd also let my dogs come along with me with me so the bigger ones could run around. (They were immune to being chased by Pasado due to their being "old news.") But I carried Charlie Bear, our tiny Chihuahua. There were many nights when I'd be cussing and yelling as I held Charlie Bear and tried to pick up an increasingly larger, squealing, Apples, without tripping on her leash, while being followed closely by llamas, emus, and Pasado, heads low in a stalking fashion.

Eventually Apples became "naughty", which simply means she started doing what was natural for a pig. Her instincts told her to root around in the yard, pull the siding off the house in the same spot the goats had previously, and even lay cuddled up against a basement window (breaking it). I was in another part of the basement when this happened and could not for the life of me figure out why it sounded like Apples was in the house. By then she didn't fit through the doggie door. I followed her squeal to the laundry room where I found her entire head looking down at me from the ground-level window. I was grateful she hadn't cut herself on the glass.

Our house had so many wounds and lesions due to animals; it was obvious we would have to raze it if we ever wanted to sell our property in the future. (Seven years later, after building the house we live in now on the same property, the old house was pushed into its own basement and buried.) We decided Apples was big and old enough to live in the "middle-sized" pasture was (about half an acre) where we kept the six pot-bellied pigs we had rescued over the years.

At first I was worried about Apples, hoping she wouldn't be hurt by the older, and still bigger, pigs. But it became obvious in no time that she was cool with her new surroundings, and was taking big advantage of them. While she had been eating a limited amount of food prior to the move from our yard, she was now getting as much as she wanted because she not only ate her rations, but the others' as well! I began feeding Apples more than enough to fill her up on one end of the pasture, then ran really fast to the far end of the pasture to feed the pot-bellied pigs their rations, hoping they ate quickly enough to avoid losing food to Apples.

With housing adjusted, Apples continued to grow and grow. I had spayed her as a piglet and didn't know how much it would affect her weight. It probably enhanced her growth rather than inhibited it. She took over the pasture and became popular with visitors. Her pasture ran along the busy county highway; so I often saw cars slow down when the pigs were out mucking about or eating. If we had spare apples in the fall I could go out on the deck and yell "Aaaaaaaappppples!" and she would come running from the far end of the pasture to the end nearest our house. I'd then start throwing apples to her from the deck, just a few dozen yards away. Sometimes an apple wouldn't make it to her and she'd get frustrated trying to get it through the fence. I would usually give in and walk all the way over to get it for her. Then she would savor a good back scratch and face rub. She even shook her back leg like a dog or cat when I scratched in her ears.

Apples continued to grow for more than a year. Her weight was such that she would lean against the fence (yes, the inappropriate chain-link) and stretch it out, creating an opening that she could later get her head through. She did this all along the fence that ran along the highway. Erosion under the fence got to the point that I needed to have several yards of dirt delivered to fill it in. I spent many hours with the shovel and wheelbarrow, going back and forth between the dirt pile and fence, thinking about that naughty, naughty, naughty "little" pig, who I still adored.

Sadly, as she grew, Apples' legs became sore. She would limp periodically on one foreleg then the other, and then be fine. But when I noticed the fact that she no longer ran out for treats, I knew she wasn't feeling as good as she once had. She could make the trip over, but at a walk, then at a limpy walk, then not at all.

Apples had been brought into this world to do one of two things: She was to be raised for several months and "finished" to a yummy, meaty body condition and butchered, having spent most of her life crowded in a barn or yard with hundreds of others. Or, she was to be raised for farrowing, possibly spending her life in a box she couldn't even turn around in, making babies for up to four years before being forced into a truck and shipped to a slaughter house. She was bred for food production for people, not for running and playing. Strong legs were not necessary, so they were not part of what had been bred into her through her DNA.

As she worsened, I began to worry about her euthanasia. How much solution would I need for the injection? How much sedative would I need beforehand? I never perform a euthanasia without heavily sedating the animal first, unless of course the animal is utterly calm or not fully conscious already. But there was another way, a faster way, a she-won't-know-what-happened-to-her way. A gun shot. I have a neighbor who owned large caliber guns. But I knew he would need to be educated on how to shoot a pig in such a way that it is quick and therefore humane. But that was a lot to ask. I also thought about how hard it would be to get her into the vehicle used by the service that performs animal cremation service.

Noting the environmental impact as well when making this decision, I realized it would take an awful lot of energy for a cremation that wasn't really necessary.

This is where I took my thinking a step further. Having decided the quick way would be better for Apples, I realized there would be no chemicals in her body to prevent her from being useful after death; her meat would be edible.

Now, I may be dividing you readers into two groups: The "Duh, of course you should eat her! She's a pig!" and the "You've got to be freaking crazy! She was a pet!!" groups.

I started talking to folks who understood me enough not to be surprised when I asked, "Do you know anyone who knows how to shoot a pig humanely, then take it away for use as food?" Jim, the man who coincidentally delivered the dirt for the fence, said he "just may know someone."

Sure enough I got a phone call, not even an hour after mentioning it to Jim, from a gentleman who said he was interested in helping me, and perhaps helping himself as well. My heart was in my throat, and I obsessed for the next 24 hours, talking to people, emailing them, calling them. Was this sick? Or was it totally logical?

In my mind, it was pretty much a coin toss. I finally called the gentlemen back. I was kind of assuming he was just someone who wanted the free meat and didn't give a crap about anything else. I almost hoped this to be the case, so I could say "no" to the selfish creep and change my mind. As it turned out, he was a 78 year old former pig farmer who had done this many times. I gave him two strict requirements: that he do his job with the gun perfectly! He said he could. And that he not force her to walk. He had to do it wherever she happened to be lying at the time. He said he would.

He came by with his son, and met Apples. By now she was grumpy; she laid about most of the time but still enjoyed being scratched. The man said she was easily 500 pounds or more. Though he kept referring to Apples as "it," I knew he was sensitive to the fact that she not be distressed and that I really loved that pig.

It had been rainy and the man planned to come the following week when the mud dried up. But after another one of his sons said he could help, they returned soon after the first visit. They were ready to do it. Apples was ready. I was not. I looked at the three men who had everything they needed to do what I had asked, just as I instructed. I was not one of those things they needed. Having just come back from giving Apples a good back scratch, I chose not to go back for one last good-bye. I could feel the overwhelming sadness inside me, and feared she might be able to sense something odd was going on. I did however watch from the window of our house. To this day I am not sure I'm glad I did. Within 30 minutes the men had taken Apples away, leaving only the impression of her body in her favorite spot as evidence that she had just been there.

I didn't ask the man for money, even though I knew he was getting a bargain. He did a job I didn't want to do myself, saved some pollution from being put into the air, and saved me quite a bit of money for sedatives and euthanasia drugs, and cremation as well. We both felt it was a fair exchange.

That pasture has been used by many other animals since Apples. Happily, the dirt I put in along the base of the fence is still there. I seeded it with wildflowers shortly after Apples died. They are really pretty during the summer; because of them it will always be Apples' pasture.

(Note: When the men and Apples were gone ,Kirsten asked "What are they going to do with her?" I hadn't explained ahead of time and worried she would be upset. Hesitantly, I said "Well, they *might* eat her." She cracked me up when she replied "But I want her. I love pork sandwiches!" Kirsten has been a devoted vegetarian since 2015 and finds it hard to believe she ever said this.)

Another Almost-Fatal Attraction

Let me set the scene for you:

One Monday morning in late winter I was getting ready for work, Kirsten was getting ready for school, and Torben was preparing for his day off. We were moving about as usual, the dogs getting more and more excited, because whenever Torben or I have a day off, the dogs get an earlier and longer walk than usual. Torben had put his boots on and walked into the living room.

"There's something in my boot," he said.

"Huh, weird," I said.

"I think something is biting me!"

"It's a spider," I said. "Yep. Bet it's a spider."

He sat down. "Ouch, it really hurts."

"Spider. Seriously. I bet it's a spider. Ahhhhhhh, I'm not looking."

Yes, I am scared of big spiders. It is very embarrassing and something I am slowly desensitizing myself to, even going so far as to adopt a tarantula from the Iowa City shelter years ago. (Would you believe the aquarium and tarantula were left on the curb at the end of the school year by college kids who were moving out?) The pet tarantula lasted only a week. I couldn't even feed it. Couldn't even watch Torben feed it. I just got so creeped out. I don't think my fear is completely irrational; I once put my bare feet into my rubber boots when I felt pain. I took the boot off, tipped it up-side-down and saw with horror a very, very, very large spider plop out. I think I blacked out because I still don't know what became of the spider. But even though I am scared of them I also don't want to kill them. Torben usually performs that task, whisking the spider up with his hand, sometimes grossing me out by offering to eat it, then tossing it outside. I feel like barfing just thinking about it.

Okay, so we all now know big spiders creep me out. Back to Torben in pain:

"Ouch, it really does hurt!"

I was about to walk into the bedroom to get away from the huge spider that I was certain was in his boot and would soon be crawling around our home, when, out of morbid curiosity, I turned to look. Torben had just removed his boot. At the end of his big toe was a flapping brown bat.

It was quite surreal, remembering the scene now. But the moment I saw it I didn't think, "Oh, poor Torben!" or "Oh my! A bat! How crazy is that?" All I could think was, "Man, we failed." The reason for my reaction is a story that starts 72 hours earlier.

A local shelter will once in a while entrust us with a bat that a homeowner found flying around in his home. At this time of year, bats are sleeping in crawl spaces and attics and such, enjoying the 40-something degree temps, huddled together, conserving their energy stores. Once in a while one may wake up, fly around a bit, then rearrange itself in the group and go back to sleep. On the other hand, it may accidentally end up in the living quarters of a home. Surprised homeowners typically freak out and either kill it or take it to animal control to be killed so it can be tested for rabies. I find this fact rather sad for bats because less than 3% of the bats tested in Iowa in the past decade actually have had rabies. If a bat is in your home, and it hasn't touched you, your chances of getting rabies are essentially zero. BUT, I know rabies is fatal, and I see why people freak out. I just hate mosquitoes and know the cute-little-flying-fuzzy-mouse-vampire-looking things love them, and need a chance to do their job.

This particular bat, I'll call Bootsie, was somewhat asleep when we got him, and had been kept cool to prevent his instinct to wake up to spring. Unfortunately, on day two he was scratching around quite a bit. When that happens, you have to start feeding the bat. Bootsie enjoyed a meal of "super worms," those gross, mealworm-looking things you may have seen people eating on the TV show *Fear Factor*. Our plan was to put together supplements the following day (to add to the worms) and get Bootsie through the rest of the winter. Bootsie ate surprisingly well, grabbing each worm with his little claws, eating it like a kid eats an ice-cream cone: bite, lick, lick, lick, bite, lick, lick, lick....

Here is where Torben and I failed Bootsie. We couldn't locate our screened cage. The screen is important because it won't damage the bat's wings if it flaps around, and it is something the bat can cling to, yet not escape. But we did have a rodent cage with bars less than a centimeter apart. We put Bootsie into the rodent cage when he had eaten his fill. We then put the cage in our bedroom (cats don't go in there, so couldn't bother him), and went to sleep ourselves.

Needless to say, Bootsie had squeezed out of the cage and flown around before resting comfortably in Torben's boot.

So we failed Bootsie terribly. Not using the proper cage was a mistake.

At this point you might be thinking, "Oh my God Jenni, what about rabies? Torben could have rabies now!" That thought did enter our minds early on. I have been receiving rabies immunizations regularly due to the work I do, so was not afraid for myself when feeding Bootsie, or pulling his little mouth off Torben's toe. Torben, on the other hand, had received only one immunization more than a decade ago. I didn't like that at all. He didn't worry much at first.

The morning of the bat-flapping-wildly-on-Torben's-toe Incident I went to work and pondered the situation. Torben didn't want to kill the bat to have it tested. I didn't either, but........

I had noticed Bootsie didn't eat well after the boot incident (I used a worm to help get him off the sock). I kept picturing his little body in the tip of Torben's boot getting squished. Bootsie had been able to squeeze to less than a cm wide, so he didn't need much space in the boot. But I still wondered "Is Bootsie going to live anyway?"

Normal sane people would have taken that little sucker to the lab immediately, but that night Torben and I were still pondering. I was worrying about Torben and I could tell he was thinking about it too, asking me things like: What are the chances the bat had rabies? When is it too late for him to get shots?

That evening I decided to take Bootsie in the next day for testing. After Torben went to bed I googled the Hygienic Lab on the UI Oakdale campus and printed the necessary forms.

At this point in the story I have a confession to make to Torben. The rest of you can skip to the next paragraph.

Torben, remember when I told you I had checked Bootsie on Tuesday morning and found him dead? I lied. He was sleeping. I looked at him and said to myself, "Gee that is a fricking cute little guy. How perfect and precious those wings are, the fuzzy body, the little ears and claws...... But I guess I like Torben just a tad bit more." I apologized to Bootsie and put him into a box and drove him to the lab.

As I started writing this story, on the following Friday, I still didn't know the results of the lab test. Yet I feel confident we would, in the future, behave as sane people do and both go in for our rabies titer test. which (The test essentially tells you if you have antibodies in your blood that could combat a rabies infection.) And we would get post-exposure injections for rabies should the test be positive and our titers low.

I sit here uneasy about how different Torben's and my thought processes are from probably 99% of the population, yet know they are just natural for the two of us. We worry about the animal, then ourselves. I am not sure why, but hope our thinking is just a circuitous neural pathway that is much longer than the thought process of a typical human being. The end result is the same. A person was bit by a bat. The bat had to be euthanized and tested for rabies. Duh. But our brains have all kinds of other "things" sprinkled in, stops our neurons have to make, before getting to the same conclusion.

I'm not sure if that is pathology or not. Maybe someone can tell me.

(Note: Bootsie was negative for rabies.)

Stinky Cats No One Could Love...
Except Just About Everybody

There is a large cats-only sanctuary in northern Iowa that I work with on and off. The founders and main caretakers are a wonderful couple of ladies who devote everything they have to the animals, going so far as to convert a childhood home into a main cat facility. I met them around 2003 when I used to drive my mobile clinic the 100 miles north to spend the day working on the injuries and ailments the few hundred (yes hundred) cats in residence.

They and I had an ongoing joke. It goes something like this:

Them (aka The Ladies): "Jenni, we have a horrendously injured cat, and we wonder if you can fix him. "

Me: "Let's see him." I then take a look and in my head, I'm thinking *Oh my God! No freaking way can I help this poor thing. What the heck do they think I am, a miracle worker?* Then I calmly say to them, "Hmm, I'll see what I can do."

We went through that scenario with three amazing kitties who all lived at least long enough to fully recover from the procedures I did, and to make many people fall completely in love with them.

Bradley was the first. He was a stray; both of his back legs were broken, one at the knee, and the other below it. Both were open fractures, and he had been walking on the broken ends of his tibias, packing dirt and whatnot up the center of them. He was so infected and stinky that it was hard to think of anything else when near him. Yet as is often the case, he had a loving personality. He thanked The Ladies constantly for their food, warmth, and safety by rubbing his head up to them and purring as they held him. It was as though he had no consciousness of those back legs of his.

I had seen cats previously with almost identical injuries. I had euthanized all of them as they were semi-feral, either trapped or captured using a net in barns or sheds. By the time I met Bradley, I had learned that not all cats are good candidates for repair, and that I shouldn't put my ego before my desire to help greater numbers of cats who had problems much easier to remedy. But in Bradley's case, I could see why his personality tipped the scales for The Ladies. He just did not care that he was broken!

At first I thought about removing the legs at the knees and running threaded pins up the center of his femurs, leaving about an inch or so sticking out on which he could walk, like peg legs. However, at the time, I didn't know if that was something that had ever been done, not that that always stops me. I just wasn't 100% sure what size pin I could run up the bone that would not slide further up the leg as he walked. Today I think I would be brave enough to do it, especially now that I have seen videos of cats that have had exactly that done by other vets. (Oh hindsight, you're so 20/20!)

So I did the best I could to provide suitable ends to his bones that would be blunt enough to prevent poking sharply into the tissue. I then had to remove so much infected skin that I didn't think there would be enough to cover the bone and muscle "padding." I also had to make the incision away from the surface that touched the ground when he walked. The surgery was a success; after a bit of recovery time, Bradley went home to The Ladies a new man.

The fullness of this cat's personality can only be grasped when you know that he immediately introduced himself to the other cats in his building at the sanctuary before taking charge of the whole place. He even got his own article in the sanctuary's newsletter. He was an unbelievably fat, black, long-haired cat who greeted folks as they entered "his" building. Bradley was so happy and loved, you couldn't help but smile when you met him. I can't wipe the dumb smile off my face right now thinking about him.

Then there was Trameel. He had been at the sanctuary a short while before I met him. Again, my first thought was not that I should try to save him, but that he was suffering and should be put down. He was actually bad enough that I wasn't shy about mentioning euthanasia. Once again, The Ladies seemed to know what I didn't yet know, that he believed he was just too cool a cat to ignore. Trameel had severe weakness in both rear legs and was fecal and urine incontinent. I suspected it was due to a tail avulsion. This is a common injury in cats whose tails are yanked so hard (by a person, or under a car tire while they're running) that the nerves and ligaments of the tail pull hard enough on the nerves and ligaments coming from the spine to create serious inflammation.

Sometimes the trauma heals and resolves the side-effects, but if not, the urinary and bowel incontinence leads to life-threatening problems. The bladder loses its ability to tell itself to relax the sphincter. So, despite a full bladder and muscles in the bladder trying to squeeze it empty, the "door" just doesn't open. When the pressure builds to a critical point, it empties, but never entirely. The urine gets stagnant, and infected, leading to kidney failure. Trameel smelled like he wasn't far from this. Furthermore, the repeated dribbling of the infected urine had caused scaling of his perineum and legs. On the bright side, he never felt a thing. Nerve damage meant he had no sensation in his skin back there, so the frequent washings The Ladies provided never bothered him. But the infection was getting to him.

So I've done the brief anatomy lesson. Now let me be frank. His rear end looked like a bloody kitchen sponge with oozing tracts erupting from its surface. The constant scalding and infection scarred and deformed him to the point where he no longer had his "boy parts." Urine was seeping from some open wounds around the usual location. I essentially had to find what I could and make him as normal as possible, cutting in the area where his penis should have been, carefully removing layer upon layer of dead tissue, and hoping to find a happy little penis peeking out of the decay. It's a bit like taking the top off a deep well and seeing, way down below, the face of the person who had been trapped there. Happily, I did find that little face, and reconstructed, the best I could, the tissue around it so it would not be covered, yet not be totally exposed.

Amazingly, again, Trameel did great. Unfortunately, he had to have help urinating by having his bladder squeezed. But he now had one place he did it from, not several, and it was much tidier. He was on a schedule of antibiotics, as he was still prone to infections; but he ended up putting on enough weight that I didn't recognize him months later. He was just one of the many tabbies running around. Sadly, we bought him only two more years of life. But I was proud that yet another almost impossible case did so well, and made so many people happy, and gave Trameel better months in the end than he had been enduring before.

Finally, there was Hot Rod. He was our "Wormie Kitten" (a.k.a. The Grub by Kirsten), not for the reasons many readers might think, but because it suited his appearance. Hot Rod had similar problems as Trameel, but his were congenital, or else had occurred very shortly after birth. Besides the incontinence, his useless back legs were deformed, rigid, and dragged through whatever he encountered along the way. Hot Rod was a tiny 8 week old orange kitten when I met him. What a personality this little guy had! Some sort of knowing look in his eyes made you feel like he was studying your face or something. He used his front legs to scoot anywhere he wanted; not knowing his rear end was a complete catastrophe. The constant dragging, urine scalding, and multiple daily cleanings had removed a significant amount of skin. Again, there was no normal anatomy to consider, and should I mention the smell?

Anyway, little Hot Rod underwent bilateral rear leg amputations, rotational skin grafts, and urethrostomy (meaning I removed what remnants of penis remained after all the dead tissue was removed and made him pee like a girl). You would think, after such an extensive and lengthy surgery under anesthesia, he would recover slowly. Not Wormie Kitten, who woke up and started gobbling down his canned food only hours later, purring as he went. It was unbelievable! Though he had sensation in his rear legs, he never let on that he hurt. Immediately after surgery I bandaged his rear end in such a way that he could pee and poop (with assistance), then covered that with a fairly tight, clean sweat sock. He looked like a glow worm toy you used to see advertised on TV in the 90s, just without the light in the butt. Not expecting him to move much, I just left him in a box in the living room, thinking he'd stay put like anyone else would after such a major procedure. But the little guy pulled himself out, and climbed up the back of a couch and down the other side the NIGHT of his surgery!

The only time Wormie complained was when I squeezed his bladder to empty it, which needed to be done several times a day. This prevented the buildup of pressure in the bladder, which would then damage the kidneys, diminish bladder tone, and predispose him to urinary infections. Due to scarring after surgery, I had to heavily sedate him twice more to widen his urethra and make it exit in such a way that it wouldn't have direct contact with the ground should his sock come off.

When it came to pooping, he did this himself. It meant changing many socks, but we had plenty. My house isn't immune to the black hole that seems to separate pairs and take mates away. Every time he soiled one I threw it in the wash and stuck another on. Pretty soon, very nice people were also giving me socks, thanks to a note in the sanctuary newsletter. With so many socks coming in, I could actually just toss them in the trash and not worry about washing the stinky little things.

But the most wonderful part of having Wormie was his companionship with a little chick that had literally been dumped into the open window of my van one night. Yes, I got up one morning, went out to my vet van, crack and found a little yellow chick. Actually, I *heard* the chick. I then had to hunt for it, following the faint peeps. I finally found it up in the mysterious area of wires and things just above where a passenger in the front seat would put his feet.

Chickie and Wormie were inseparable. They slept together in the bathtub at night, and ran around free in the house during the day. On days I worked, they went in the van with me; I kept them in one of the built-in cages just above the cab. While doing surgeries at the back of the van, I could look forward and see them huddled together, sometimes even see Wormie licking Chickie. While loose in my house, Chickie would have been easy pickings for my other cats who liked to go birding, but living with Wormie gave Chickie a real empowered, tough-guy attitude that scared all the cats away. I laughed so hard when Chickie would realize she somehow had ended up on the opposite side of a room from Wormie, and she would suddenly run at him. Then, just before reaching him, she'd leap up and peck him between the eyes. This would start a big, rough battle, almost looking like Wormie would finally take Chickie apart, and then it'd end in a big love hug with licking, cuddling, and purring.

Wormie stayed with us a month before being ready to go back to The Ladies at the sanctuary, where he continued to do well, yet still needed his bladder expressed daily. Many months later, after developing another urinary infection, he declined quickly and had to be put down, I assume due to kidney complications. I was no longer making regular trips up to that sanctuary, so wasn't the primary veterinarian. I was happy to know he was a popular and happy boy during his stay there.

Sadder to me, though, was the loss of Chickie, yet another freak accident. The day Wormie left, our family had an event to attend, so I locked Chickie up in the bathroom as usual. I made a fatal mistake, however, and did not close our toilet. When I came home that night and went in to check on him, I was shocked and saddened to find him drowned. I can't help but feel like such an idiot at times! However, I've never made that mistake again if we leave animals, no matter what kind, in our bathroom.

Wormie and Chickie were two tiny little specimens who seemed almost perfect in their imperfections. Their short lives sank in and stayed with me. When they were gone, it was that much harder.

Wormie and Chickie, Trameel and Bradley are examples of wonderful animals I'd never have worked with in a million years if I were still in an everyday pet practice. I've learned a tremendous amount medically, and have examples to draw upon when wondering whether putting out that extra effort is worth it. I thank The Ladies so much for sending me those impossible cases. I can't wait for the next one.

Charlie the Goose

It is interesting how quickly a quiet Sunday can be turned completely around with the minor suggestion of an animal in need.

One Sunday early in the fall of 2012, I was probably relaxing by scooping litter boxes and feeding some sort of animal, when I noticed I had received a text from Jane, a local animal rescuer. Her text was about a goose at a local golf club who had been walking around on the course for most of the summer with a broken wing. It seemed otherwise all right, just couldn't fly. People had made half-hearted attempts to catch it but without the urgency of winter no one tried especially hard. Jane's people were now aware of it and were intent on catching it, as autumn can turn quickly to winter in this region. Could I help out? (When Jane texted me it usually meant the group had caught the animal already and needed me to tend to it, and keep it for a day or two......or forever.) This time Jane simply asked if I would take it in and see if I could help it. I responded that I would. She in turn responded that they would try to capture it and get it to me by 4:00 that afternoon.

I pushed the goose to the back of my mind since I didn't need to act on it for the moment. However, shortly after Torben returned from his Sunday jog I mentioned to him a goose would be coming around 4:00. He asked why so late, and I told him it was because it was still running around the golf course and had to be caught. His response was, "Why don't we just go out ourselves and get it now?"

Even though, in the back of my mind, I wondered how the heck the two of us (and Kirsten, almost 8 years old) would catch it when no one had been able to all summer, I simply said, "Okay". It was a beautiful sunny day. Why not? I gathered blankets and the three of us set off.

On the way to the golf course, only about ten miles north of our home in a rural area, I remembered Jane had mentioned a golf tournament was going on that day. Hmm, I thought, that's probably why Jane's rescue group was not going to attempt to catch it until later. It also occurred to me that perhaps we should have contacted the golf course before coming. Oh heck, we would deal with it when we got there. After introducing ourselves to the young staff folks, who were very nice, they gave us a golf cart and we set off to the area where the goose was last seen.

I am not a golfer, never will be. Walking out of the clubhouse to get into the cart, I felt absolutely out of place. I was dressed in torn jeans and t-shirt and here I was, hanging around with all these more conservative and tidily dressed folks. I didn't feel inferior, just different. Torben still had on his sweaty jogging shorts and shirt. Kirsten just looked cute as usual. We went down the path to the large pond we had been directed to, where we quickly spotted the goose all alone on the bank. The wing dragged and seemed to slow it down.

Despite being hindered by his wing on land, we quickly found he had no trouble speeding along once in the water, which of course is where he went once we parked our cart near him and climbed out. We looked on with a combination of amazement (at his ability) and a bit of disappointment (for us). It was a big pond. He was a fast swimmer. At this point Torben just took off his shirt and shoes and waded in. Mind you, it was Iowa in the fall. Despite the sunny day, the water was very cold. Not only that, Torben's sudden drop to neck level only a few yards in, meant that it was deep! I had no idea a golf course needed such big and deep ponds. How were the golfers supposed to get their balls back? Torben couldn't touch bottom shortly after going out to the middle. For the longest time he just swam around, lurking, following the goose, looking like a crocodile closing in on its prey. The biggest difference was the fact that the goose was completely aware he was there, and Torben was not submerging for an underwater surprise attack. Wimp.

While Torben paddled after the goose, it made quiet little honks as it led him back and forth from one end of the pond to the other. I kept following them along the shore, which did not have a nice gentle grassy bank, but rather had those big rocks you see in ditches to help keep soil from eroding. I stumbled my way over them, wondering how long this could go on, and thinking we must have looked really lame to anyone watching. Kirsten just sat quietly in the cart, watching, likely wondering (not for the first time) how she had landed parents like this.

After what felt like a very long time, Torben called for me to move the cart, pointing to the opposite side of the pond from where I was standing at the time. I wasn't sure why, but dutifully stumbled up the bank and plopped down next to Kirsten. It was then that I realized I had never driven a golf cart before. So when the thing didn't start after I turned the key, I freaked out. I was out of my comfort zone. I tried over and over before finally putting my foot on the "gas" pedal. It started and I drove it to the end of the pond where the goose was heading. It was clear that Torben was sick of following the thing and decided to chase it onto shore.

When I reached the bank where the goose was headed, I was relieved that it would have trouble scrambling up the bank (like I had) and be easy to catch. That little sucker flopped his way up the bank just as I was leaping out of the still rolling cart. (Don't worry. Kirsten had the wheel.) He ran, very fast, down the long length of dark green golf grass that has a name I do not know (fairway? lane? runway? should I care?). I sprinted faster than I had since high school, over THREE decades earlier, chasing it finally into some trees, having to stumble through weeds and low branches the goose was able to duck under. Just before he was to the opposite edge of the trees, on his way out to clear space again, he stumbled too. That was when I was able to grab him.

On my way back toward the pond, I could hear Kirsten laugh and laugh and laugh several hundred yards away. I was breathing hard and hesitantly looked around to see who had seen the 47 year old woman chasing down a crippled goose, and having trouble doing so. Thankfully there were no golfers in the immediate area, only my daughter. Feeling pleased with the job, I returned to the cart and wrapped the goose up in a sheet before Torben drove us back to the club house. On the way, we passed a spot where some guy was teeing off. Torben politely stopped and turned off the cart so the guy could take his turn. After he did, but before the second guy took his swing, we started up and drove off, hearing, "Hey! We're teeing off here!" At first we thought the guy yelling was a jerk; mad because we didn't wait for him despite the fact that he hadn't even put his tee in the ground. But after thinking about it, maybe we weren't supposed to drive along the big long dark green length of grass they were hitting the ball down. I don't care enough about golf to find out if that was the reason why.

By the time we got home we had named the goose Charlie and declared him to be a boy, even though I had not officially sexed him. Turning him over and probing him was not a priority. A new sex designation could be made at a later time. He was mad as heck, pecking and flapping once the sheet had been loosened. His wing was obviously broken high on the humerus. The firm swelling at the broken ends and mobility of the site indicated it had tried to heal without success.

The following Wednesday I took Charlie to an Iowa City veterinary hospital for radiographs. We quickly found he had a multiple-fragment fracture of the humerus, spanning most of the bone. Some of the pieces had healed together at an odd angle at the ends of the bones, but many were still "lying around." I sent the radiographs to the vet specialists in this area who said there was little (some, but not much) hope of him being repaired well enough to be released.

The following Sunday, only a week after we'd caught him, we anesthetized him and removed his wing. I was stressed because birds are very tricky when it comes to anesthesia. Prep is also kind of creepy because instead of shaving hair at the site that will be operated on, the feathers needed to be plucked! Pulling the feathers out of a live bird is trickier than it seems. It is easy to accidentally tear the skin. Even though I feel I did a great job of removing the wing and not letting Charlie die during surgery, I scolded myself for being wimpy and not taking more of those tiny downy feathers off. They ended up being of little consequence, but I made a mental note to do a better job should I ever do another bird surgery, which I knew I would.

Once awake and up from anesthesia, Charlie was much more agile and quick. I think he had been hurting much more before the surgery than I realized at the time. I imagined how painful it must have been for him when scrambling up the pond bank, or trying to ditch me in the weeds at the golf course.

Thanks to Lilly, a master wildlife rehabilitator from an area near Cedar Falls, I was hooked up with a woman who had an ideal site for Charlie to live out the rest of his life along with other Canada geese. She and her husband own several acres with a pond surrounded by trees. They keep the pond aerated to prevent freezing over in winter. They care for several flightless ducks and geese.

Less than three weeks after the adventure with Charlie began, I was driving an hour and a half north to Cedar Falls with him in a large crate in the back of my van. He was still wild, not wanting anything to do with me, and totally unappreciative, exactly the way I prefer wildlife to be. Letting wildlife go was easier if they just did not give a darn about me. It didn't hurt my feelings.

When we arrived at the property I was thrilled. It was the type of property I wouldn't mind owning, out away from other houses, with a large pond, and hidden. The woman and her husband were very nice. We walked down to the beach where they fed the birds. She called them and tossed corn out. A half dozen geese, many with names, swam over from a small island or sand bar in the middle of the pond. It was at this point I opened Charlie's crate. He quickly walked out, stood and stared at the others for a while, then swam out towards them. Linda predicted he would suddenly start bathing himself vigorously, which he did, dunking over and over. There was a little bit of a scuffle before they all went back together to join the rest of the flock. I could keep an eye on Charlie because his bright white feathers that would otherwise be covered by his wing were easily visible.

I was so happy for him.

But alas, I couldn't stay long. I had to get back home to meet the newest patient being dropped off at our place. A local park employee had picked up an adult white pelican that was very weak and dragging a wing. He would be my first pelican and I had no idea what to expect. That would be another story.

Eating Crow

I did a stupid thing today. I saved a wild animal on the road. Why stupid? It was because of how I went about it. I did it in a way that made me say something I've heard my son, Joseph, say more than a few times: "Mom! What the .... is wrong with you? You wanna get killed for an animal?" Before you start thinking Joseph isn't caring and compassionate, I have to tell you that when he says those words, he is absolutely right, maybe 90% of the time. He usually yells them as I am slamming on my brakes or swerving into the ditch to avoid, say, even a toad. I have a way of compartmentalizing too well when I see a hurt animal, so much so that nothing else exists. But today, even I am saying, "What the .... is wrong with me!?"

Here's the scene: It was February 3, 2015, a bitterly cold Midwestern day. We had just had a huge dumping of snow two days prior. The trees, fences, and houses were still heavily covered with the stuff. I was driving Kirsten to school in time for her 7:30 a.m. tech club meeting, taking our usual back road, which is very curvy and hilly. As a responsible driver, I drove slower than usual, didn't stare at how beautiful the trees looked, or play with the radio. I just drove, watching ahead of me.

Shortly after getting to the curviest section of the road, I saw a crow sitting in the middle of it. I slowed down, assuming it would fly away as I drove by. It flapped its wings as we passed. I looked in the rear-view mirror and realized it hadn't flown away and was just sitting there again. Suddenly my brain switched to *hurt-animal-tunnel-vision-mode*.   I   immediately stopped and backed up, which actually was difficult because the windows were frosted up. No surprise, given all the warm breath coming from me, Kirsten, and the three big dogs who *had* to come for the ride, and the walk that would follow since it was my day off. I opened my window and saw that as I backed up to the bird, it hopped quickly into the ditch, and crowed. Wait, roosters crow. The crow cawed, I think. Whatever, it was a raucous noise that carried on for several seconds.

Without thinking beyond the cry of a hurt bird, I drove straight into the opposite ditch, sinking the car into snow well past its bumpers. Fortunately, I was able to pull out of it, and then parked. I stumbled out of the car and into the ditch near the crow, which by now was running into the woods. I was able to grab it when it got tangled in some weeds. After the catch, I turned and began walking through the waist deep snow. As I crawled out of the ditch, I got the first inkling of my stupidity when I looked up the road, where my van was parked and still running.

First, I was parked in the center of an icy road at the bottom of a hill and had left my door open. Not only was parking there stupid, but stopping suddenly and backing up was as well. Second, the open driver's-side door allowed Mumma dog to get out. She was standing dead center in the oncoming traffic lane. I trotted over, yelling at Mumma, "Go Home! Go Home!" which is my command for the dogs to get into the car. She did. She happily jumped back in and I followed, crow in my arms.   As I pulled away, without putting on my seatbelt, a school bus drove past us from the opposite direction. If you knew that bus driver, you'd know it was speeding along with momentum that couldn't be stopped by a cement truck, let alone little old Mumma Dog or me, with or without the crow.

I now felt sick to my stomach that I had been so careless. But wait! There was more. I drove with one hand while holding the crow with the other. I asked Kirsten to hold the crow. This entire time she had been sitting in the back seat looking at my phone, perhaps not even realizing the drama going on around her.

"Just hold his wings down. His claws are scratchy but your coat will keep him from hurting you."

No sooner did I say this than the crow bit her.

"He bit me!" she said and immediately held him up for me to grab.

As I reached out blindly with my right hand behind my seat, the crow took hold of my finger, the fleshy part of the tip of my right index finger, and held on like a vice.

"He's biting you!" Kirsten cried.

"I'm Okay. It's Okay." I said, all the while amazed at how much it really hurt. By now I had put on my seatbelt, and kept driving, while the crow continued to stay clamped down on the skin of my finger.

As I drove, I apologized to Kirsten and gave thanks that he wasn't still attached to Kirsten's finger instead of mine. When it became apparent he was not letting go anytime soon, I got to thinking about something most people don't worry about. How much do I really need that part of my body? I mean, I knew the worst he could do was take the large piece of skin he was biting down on, but it was the index finger on my dominant hand, a hand I use for surgery. I knew the answer, because I had asked myself the same question before, when I was bit by the timber rattlesnake several years ago. Back then I wondered, "Could I live without my entire right index finger?" The answer was "Yeah, I suppose I could." If I had to choose not to have a finger on my right hand, the three I *couldn't* live without are my thumb, middle and ring fingers. Perhaps a tad morbid, but that is what I've decided. Asking myself theoretical questions of all types is a favorite thing to do if my brain wanders.

The crow kept hold of my finger. I was afraid that if I pulled away he might bite Kirsten. I finally slowed the car way down. (Stop? No, that would have made too much sense.) I quickly turned back to pry his beak open with my left hand only to have him clamp down on the skin of my knuckle, this time making it bleed. As I took him from Kirsten, he mercifully let go before sitting quietly on my lap the rest of the drive to school.

When we arrived, I wrapped the crow tightly in one of the many blankets I have in the car and slid the bundle into a five-gallon pail that was on the floor of the passenger side. I said my goodbyes to Kirsten, and drove off. At this point the feeling set in that I was a horribly careless mother (you're all thinking it, come on now) who needed to keep her sensible "mothering brain" (yes, I have one) functioning, despite her other, *less important*, passions. I felt horrible!

The feeling lingered at the grocery store, the gas station, and on the drive back to Sandy Beach, where I let the dogs run. I felt I had failed miserably and was thankful things turned out okay, instead of ending with a car rear-ending my van when I was parked in the middle of my lane, or Mumma dog getting hit by a car while standing in the middle of the other, or Kirsten getting a bad bite to her face......

I resolved to keep in mind the fact that this sudden tunnel-visioning happens to me, and that I need to be more realistic about my actions and expectations. I am not hopeless. It had been a very long time since I felt I was reckless while trying to deal with a road-injured animal. As I finished the drive home, I think I proved myself capable. A male cardinal was sitting alone on the road in my lane, not far from where the crow had been. I checked my rearview mirror to be sure no one was driving behind me, slowed down as I approached it and ....the bird flew away. Such an everyday idea for most people will always have to be a conscious effort for me: "Animals don't come before the safety of a mother of two children." Obvious? Duh. But I'm afraid I tend to make things harder than they need to be.

The crow had no obvious injuries I could see at first. I hoped he had been stunned by a car and just needed some time. Coincidentally, our old farm house was abandoned at that time, as our family had just moved into our new one on the same property. The old house was trashed, thanks to my turning it into the scariest haunted house ever the previous Halloween for Kirsten's annual party. I had also removed many of the windows, but the crow found a good temporary home in our first floor bathroom, where he had a view of the old back yard. I watched as he tried to hop onto the sink and then onto the shower rod, and noticed he favored a wing. Allowing myself to be bitten a few more times, I re-examined the wings and again found no obvious breaks or dislocations. I simply provided him with a little rest and a daily ration of as much food as he wanted, canned and dried dog food, shelled corn, chicken grain, and some water. No more fingers for him.

I visited the crow twice daily because he needed thawed water; the old farmhouse was not being heated anymore. Every few days I noticed him moving more fluidly, using his wings and hopping less. After about three weeks I decided to open his door, allowing him to find his way out of the bathroom, then out one of the openings where we once had windows. I would make sure he had plenty of food should he not want to leave.

The next day I did see a crow in the largest tree by the old house crowing, I mean cawing, in a loud obnoxious voice. I hadn't noticed any crows around the house on the other days, so I assumed it could be my guy. I smiled to myself and sent him a telepathic warning to behave, and wished him well. Perhaps, in his raucous way, he was saying the same to me.

Icky Bits (Part 1)

I have whined about the grossness of some aspects of my work; like feeding mice to reptiles, cleaning wounds full of maggots, doing surgery while lying in filth with my face only inches from a pig's butt. It is hard to express, though, just how some of the odd tiny little details of my days have become the norm. I often find that when I speak about these particular facts to people who are not "animal people," I sense they are thinking that it all sounds downright insane. I must admit I don't entirely disagree with those people. To me, however, those people will not be able to look back and say to themselves, "Huh, now I have done some really crazy stuff," and smile about it.

Having said that, I admit that the crazy stuff I experience is still sometimes gross. Here are a few little items I would like to share. You can be the judge as to my sanity.

The winter after having Charlie the goose, we took in another Canada goose that had been stumbling around with fishing line wrapped around its legs, and a wing. It was a ridiculously cold winter, and the poor thing was so thin, alone, and sad-looking. By the time I met him most of the line had been removed, but it was still deeply embedded into the legs, especially the one which had managed to grow tissue around the line so it was no longer visible. We found the line after we sedated the poor guy and started cutting, digging, and unwinding. It is unbelievable that fishing line can stay so strong after I don't-know-how-long it took for tissue to completely grow over it; loosening it was not an easy job.

The foot of the worst limb was cold, but heck, so was the other one. It was January for God's sake. But it didn't move in a flexible way the other one did when the goose walked. Just like Charlie, Nameless got to be in the large chain-link pen with the pond Lex the alligator used to live in. Because the pond was frozen, we put out a large warm tub of water daily in which he bathed and drank. At that time, we were still living in the old farmhouse, so I was able to watch him by just stepping out the front door onto the small porch. He was lonely, but I did not dare let him go until he healed and put on weight.

One day. while out in the yard, I was showing a gentleman the siding from our house that needed to be reattached. It was really frigid and a bit windy. We were looking at the house and the guy was talking away. Bored, I kept looking at the goose who had just gotten out of the tub and was limping around the pen. The man kept talking. I was still bored. I kept watching Nameless when all of the sudden I saw the goose take a step and keep going, leaving his bad foot behind! I stared in disbelief. Seriously, that goose's leg popped right off and was standing straight up in the air on its own. (I assume the don't-put-your-tongue-on-an-icy-flagpole caused the we foot to stick to the dry icy ground.) The goose was not hopping and stumbling. He seemed to be doing okay using his wings to help keep him upright. The whole thing went unnoticed by the man. Having no idea what he had said, yet agreeing to it, I said good-bye and that he could work on the house the next day.

I know I've done and seen gross stuff, but for some reason the sight of that still-standing leg was beyond anything I could get close to! Believe it or not, I had to have Torben go into the pen and get it. I couldn't even look at it. The experience was just so surreal it creeped me out.

The happy ending is that later that same winter it had warmed up a bit and we were able to take Nameless up to the same pond where Charlie lived. By then he was stronger, got along as well as he could, and still hated me like he should have.

My understanding is that he paired up pretty quickly with another goose and proved to be a very good flyer. He disappeared several days after arriving at his new home, no doubt putting his best foot forward and starting his new life somewhere else.

Icky Bits (Part 2)

Someone I have not mentioned yet is Lucifer, a Burmese python we had for about a decade, and who grew to be 16 feet long. As I recall, Lucifer may have been involved in a drug dealing situation before coming to us. I remember one Sunday driving to Des Moines and meeting a very young, well-tattooed and pierced couple in a crappy little hatchback car at a fast-food restaurant. It was cloudy, but fairly warm. The couple was required to get rid of their snake, so were ready to just hand him over.

Sensing distress in this young couple, and seeing a snake involved, Torben reached in his pocket, took out his wallet, pulled out a hundred dollars, and handed it to the girl. I remember being a little surprised, not because Torben hasn't been known to do things like this. As a matter of fact, I dare say I have witnessed him giving up to 100% tips to waiters and waitresses in the restaurant if he felt for some reason the person seemed really needy and had served us well. This practice is both an annoying, yet endearing, quality of his.

Still, I was a bit surprised because we had by then agreed that buying animals was not what we did. However, as Torben explained, he knew the couple was in trouble with the law, and just plain felt sorry for them.

Though Lucifer was named after the devil, he was anything but. He was always the mellowest, gentlest of giants. It was not long before Lucifer became the go-to snake when we gave talks at schools and libraries. We sometimes took him outdoors to slither around the yard for tour groups, and placed him in the arms of people standing in a row for a photo. I sometimes felt sorry for him, as he was often surrounded by twenty people, and once in a while even a dog or two. Yet he never behaved any differently outside than he did when he was in the shelter of his cage.

The most difficult part of having Lucifer was his specific food needs. Unlike the other large snakes who were happy with thawed frozen rats, Lucifer would eat nothing but rabbits. As a matter of fact, it was because of Lucifer I tried raising rabbits for a short period of time. Rabbits are expensive to buy. Getting one at a pet store could cost ten to twenty dollars. Getting them frozen from our regular company was no cheaper once you took the expensive shipping into account. We did finally receive a tip from someone who knew of a woman in Manchester, about an hour and a half north of where we lived, who raised meat rabbits.

Thanks to our new source, we could get pounds of freshly killed and frozen rabbits for a fraction of our previous cost, even when my time and gas were taken into account. The woman met me in a Walmart parking lot just outside town. It was always a short little meeting. We would recognize each other quickly because we parked in a remote part of the lot, almost behind the store. She handed me a box or two, and I handed her money. We chatted, then left.

After meeting a few times, she asked if I was interested in "extra parts." Always happy to get free food, and to help someone use up the entire body of an animal killed for food, I said sure I'd be interested. The next visit she gave me a few boxes, about 20 pounds each. of "extra parts." The boxes were labeled "heads."

"Heads?" I asked.

"Yeah, these are the heads. We don't do anything with them, though once in a while we'll give them to the dogs. We have so many we have to bury most of them."

"Um, Okay, thanks." I took them home.

I was happy to have the extra food. At the time we had Minnie and Scoopie, the coyotes, but no bear. I was not about to let my dogs have the rabbit heads, as I didn't want them lying around our yard. The more I thought about it as I drove home, I liked the idea of feeding bunny heads less and less. Later that day I told Torben about it. I don't recall him being interested one way or the other, but he did say, "Gee how nice." That was about it.

It took a long time before I actually thawed a "head" box and opened it. I surprised myself by gasping and stepping away after I opened the box and removed the plastic on top. Looking back at me through open, semi-open, and closed eyes were faces of little white rabbits. I was not hardened enough to be Okay with it. However, being the pragmatic, I bucked up and gingerly removed a couple by the ears and took them down to the coyotes. Thinking they would be thrilled to eat them immediately, I tossed the heads over the fence and then turned my own head. I didn't want to picture them flying through the air and landing on the ground. When I opened my eyes, I saw Scoopie, then Minnie slide forward to smell them. Minnie quickly ran away empty-mouthed. Scoopie, on the other, hand decided to play with her food. She immediately began to toss her bunny head into the air, finding it, then tossing it again. She ran, she frolicked, she loved the head! It was her friend. She would not eat a friend.

Disgusted with her, and with me, and with the situation, I walked back up to the house, and looked at the big box of dead bunny heads. I closed it and threw the entire thing into the garbage bin. I had another two boxes, so I knew we would not have a shortage of heads for Scoopie to play with. Days later, having forgotten about the heads, I was standing in the coyote pen, picking up litter they had dragged around and boxes they had torn apart. (I often put tasty foods into sealed boxes to give the girls fun challenges and to keep them from becoming bored.) I reached down to pick up an amorphous blob stuck to some cardboard and was shocked to see it was a still intact bunny head, minus an eye, maybe two. At that moment, I decided I would throw the other two boxes away. I was too squeamish.

However, being a procrastinator, that never happened. Those bunny heads sat in the chest freezer a while. This ended up being a good thing. Several months went by and we found ourselves rabbitless. For some reason, Lucifer had not been eating well. Torben had fed him a few rabbits, a few weeks apart, and found them uneaten. If not eaten, Torben would have to remove the rabbit and feed it to someone else before it spoiled. He was very worried about Lucifer. So every week he tried to give Lucifer another rabbit.

Eventually we ran out of frozen rabbits, there were no rabbits available from our source, and the order from the frozen rodent place would take a couple weeks. Torben had actually gone to the local pet store, bought a pet rabbit and tried it. Trouble was Lucifer ,killed it but didn't eat it.

Getting increasingly worried and crabby about the situation, Torben began moping around. He was sad the bunny had to die needlessly. We later remembered that the other weird thing about Lucifer's eating habits was that if a rabbit smelled at all like people, he wouldn't eat it. I felt reassured knowing Torben was not going to buy another pet store bunny, but we had no supply on the way.

Because I am known as a "Jenni-rigger" I began problem-solving in my head. It then hit me. We have rabbit heads. "Would he eat just a head?" I asked. Torben looked at me like I had just asked if snakes ate with a knife and fork. Okay, no heads.

But wait! We had jumbo-sized frozen rats in the freezer. I had an idea. I would suture a rabbit head onto a big rat's body. It would work!

"It won't work," Torben scowled. I couldn't hold it against him. Lucifer was like Torben's "Old Yeller."

As usual, I went ahead with my plan to prove him wrong, to prove me right, and to help Lucifer. I don't know which was more important at the time.

So I took out the rabbit head box and two giant rats. I let them thaw, then put the heads into a pail of warm water with the two rats. I wanted to be sure the rats smelled like rabbits. Once the nice pail of rabbit and rat soup had "simmered" a bit, I took out my surgical instruments. With the needle holder, thumb forceps, and suture, I tacked a rabbit head to the top of the head of each of the dead rats. As I did this, while sitting on my front porch, I thought how odd it was that I was happily humming away and sewing. I wondered if this was like the domestication of Lizzie Borden. Finally I had two "ratbits" completed. I soaked them one more time with the other thawed heads, then waited for Torben.

"It's not going to work."

"Try it."

"No."

"Try it. Why not? I worked so *hard* putting them together! "Not going to work," he said as he walked to the reptile building, carrying one of my creations with a long tongs, to avoid getting his scent on it."

I went back into the house, hoping it would work.

A few minutes later Torben came back to the house and quietly mumbled. But he was really happy. "You did it. He ate it." I was so happy and was doing a happy dance inside, but just said calmly, so as not to gloat, "Oh goody". A day or two later he fed the other hybrid animal to Lucifer with success. His fast was over. After that he went back to eating regular rabbits. Wanting to be helpful, I offered to sew more heads onto rats, but then realized what I was offering. Though I was happy it worked, and knew it was a bit of a money saver since big rats are cheaper than rabbits, I really didn't enjoy the Frankenstein act enough to make it a regular habit.

It wasn't until years later, after Lucifer had died at an advanced old age that decided to remove the remaining rabbit heads from the freezer. I had mixed emotions about it. As disgusting as they were, they had served us very well. I had taken a photo of my "ratbit" creation shortly after making it and shared it with all who would dare look at it. "See what I am willing to do for a snake," I bragged.

The photo is locked into an old broken cell phone and likely lost forever. I smile when I come across a gift that a friend made for me just a few days after I did my handiwork. It is a toy, stuffed animal rabbit head sewn onto a toy stuffed-rat. It sits upstairs with some of my prized souvenirs and will remind me when I am very old that I had dabbled a bit as a Dr. Frankenstein.

Icky (Possibly the Ickiest) Bits
(Part 3)

By now it is obvious; I am fairly Okay with handling and seeing some pretty gross stuff and I might be seen as pretty gross myself. I get it. Okay.

The fact that we order frozen rats, mice, and rabbits of varying sizes has been mentioned a few times already. Opening a box that arrives packed with dry ice is always a bummer; but I have become used to the immobilized little bodies frozen in various positions packed into Ziploc bags. The usual inventory: one adult rabbit per bag, two jumbo rats per bag, and one hundred pinkies (hairless baby mice) per bag.

My tolerance for the furred adult bodies is solid. I am quite stoic about putting them away in one of the few freezers we own specifically for them. When it comes to the littlest ones, however, those tiny little pinkies, which are only a day or so old, I have more of a problem. Two reasons, One is the mere fact that they are little babies, and that if I do look too closely at them after they've thawed, I will be able see the their last meal of milk in their little stomachs right through their transparent skin. It is sad. Then I remind myself that the company euthanizes these mice and that they were not just stuck into a freezer. So I get a grip and remind myself snakes and other reptiles need to eat. There are not enough people willing to take care of unwanted snakes. I have to do this and I can. Just buck up and stop being a baby.

Then I'm fine. I'll go days with being fine, until I get to the bottom of the clear plastic bag and see what is left behind after I've fed the last of the pinkies. Then I'm hit with Reason Two. The pinkies are so solidly frozen (below the typical household freezer) that their little legs and tails snap off their little bodies when rustled around in the bag. As a result you have several dozen soft, wet, pink little feet (toes distinguishable), and tails stuck to the side of the bag. The first time I ever had this realization I actually felt nauseous. All that was left in the bag was dismembered baby tails and toes. What do you do with those? I used to immediately throw the bag away to avoid having to look at the icky, sad little mouse bits.

But as is typically the case, with time my practical side came out and I wondered what I could do with all those little morsels. Surely they didn't need to go to waste. My answer came to me when a tiny baby snapping turtle came to us at the end of summer a couple years ago. Torben decided to fatten him up and let him go the following spring (and a fatter baby you will never find, as it turned out). I decided to put the pinkie bits in with him. There was one problem. I was not willing to pick each mouse part out one-at-a-time from the bag. So I would put some of the turtle's water into the bag, swirl the bits around, and then pour the soup back into the turtle tank.

I was too embarrassed to tell Torben I had been grossed out by the bits, so I didn't even mention how I had decided to use them. I also didn't want him to think I was doing it to make him feel guilty. He knows I have a stronger affinity for furred animals over scaled (generally speaking). Even he isn't necessarily fond of the fact that rodents need to die. But what are you going to do? When I told him about the icky bits soup I was feeding to the baby turtle, however, he told me had been doing it too. I was surprised he had never suggested it to me, but decided he may have thought the subject was too extreme, even for me.

The ones who really benefit from our soup are the little turtles. After releasing the baby snapper into the wild, too fat to pull into his shell, I thought the pinky bits had done a good job at supplementing his diet. Right now we have a small map turtle who benefits every several days, as another bag of pinkies is polished off, leaving him with nutritious soup.

So…. On those nice sunny summer days when the non-snake reptiles are fat and happy outside, the pens are not muddy, and all the furry, feathered and scaly animals are out sunning themselves, I can see it might look like our own little Sunnybrook Farm. Now you know the truth.

I've revealed the most distasteful things I have done and still do to keep animals happy and healthy and my commitment to a "waste-not" philosophy. Much of the practical, day-to-day stuff is enough to make plenty of people cringe. As uncomfortable as it can be, I just remember no one else wants most of these guys. Those who do can't have them legally. So here we are. We would transfer any of the animals to another facility if the new place were better, and the facility could come and pick them up for transport. Folks in areas of the country where finances allow for animal sanctuaries and shelters to have state-of-the-art pens and paid employees may look at what we do and feel we are inadequate. For those people I say, this is the rural Midwest. We are the best some animals have got in the entire Eastern portion of Iowa. It's that simple.

Until there is another place for them all, I will keep doing what I do. And, yes, some of it is gross.

Oh the Irony

"The Smallest Feline is a Masterpiece"

Leonardo da Vinci

The Iowa Humane Alliance of Iowa has done over 35,000 spays and neuters, mostly cats, along with dogs, rabbits, guinea pigs, rats, and even pot-bellied pigs. We have been open only since 2013, and have maintained a remarkably low complication rate. The organization is proud and more motivated than ever to help eliminate unwanted and unnecessary litters. The work of the IHA is taking pressure off local shelters and rescues that struggle with resources, and sometimes have to euthanize due to lack of space or ability to care for the sheer number of animals people bring through the doors.

The "problem" is that while I am doing everything I can to spay and neuter every cat in the state of Iowa until I can no longer do so, I am absolutely in love with the creatures I am trying to prevent from being born: KITTENS!

The irony isn't lost on me.

This morning I walked into the cat room at IHA to check in more than 30 cats. My radar immediately took me to a crate with 5 perfect little faces. It was a heavenly sight; each kitten was doing its own thing, unaware of the fact that I wanted to grab them all and run away with them. One little brown tabby sat, licking one of her paws, once in a while spreading her toes wide as if to let her little digits dry out. Two tabby brothers sat staring at me in bewilderment, while a puffy tabby-ish with white stood up crying like the little baby she was. The mostly white calico stayed asleep on her side, oblivious to the fact that I was messing with her siblings. When I opened the crate, everyone (except lazy calico) looked up at me. OH! The face of a kitten is perfection!

They were just shy of 8 weeks old, and were stunning to me. If I could do nothing but play with kittens, my days would be perfect. Instead, I cuddled them one at a time, checked them in, weighed them (all just under two pounds), and placed them into cages. They would be going under anesthesia in a few hours and the next time I was to see them, would be while they slept, under surgical lights, attached to an anesthetic machine, and ready for me to do my work. I much prefer to do kitten spays, rather than adults. First, they seem to bounce back faster. Second, they aren't fat! You have no idea how much more difficult it is to spay a cat once she has begun accumulating fat in her belly. Third, they can go to new homes and no one has to worry about them being parents in the future.

Why am I so adamant about spay/neuter? It is because I have worked at a few shelters who were high volume, open-intake organizations; this means they are willing to take in every animal that comes in.

They don't say no, which keeps people from abandoning the animals, a good thing, but because these shelters take in everyone, they run out of space quickly. Time and resources are always limited at these facilities, and when they are full beyond capacity, they cannot care properly for their charges, and so are forced to euthanize. Usually the ones euthanized are the old, the sick, or those with behavioral issues, **then** often the beautiful and healthy.

These open-intake shelters, which employee people who are committed to doing the best they can for each animal in their care, are cruelly called "kill-shelters", a term I adamantly oppose. These "Kill-shelters" are organizations that are doing their best to keep animals off the street. They also know that euthanasia is part of the deal. They do not enjoy or take lightly the need for euthanasia. Who would? I've heard time and time again folks say things like, "Oh, I could never work at a shelter. I love animals too much." Well darlings, you do **not** love animals too much. The people who love animals too much are the ones caring for them day in and day out, getting attached to them, helping them find homes, all for very little money.

If a shelter can manage a healthy and organized foster care program, it can lessen the need for euthanasia. In rural Iowa, and in other places all over the US, huge amounts of money are not tossed the way of animal shelters without having to jump through a whole lot of hoops. Donations and grants fund non-municipal shelters, meaning no one is getting rich here.

If you listened to NPR years ago when Dick Gordan had his "The Story" show, you may have heard an interview with me as part of his "Tough Jobs" series. In the segment, I explained euthanizing healthy kittens, an experience that stays emblazoned in my brain. It is a valuable image for me, especially while spaying a very pregnant cat. I know in my heart how emotionally painful it is to inject a fatal substance into a fuzzy, healthy little body. If I can euthanize a kitten before birth, I am preventing the mother from having another few stressful weeks of nursing, and preventing the need to do surgery on yet more kittens.

It all sounds callous. Believe me it is not. I've wept over the situation more times than I care to count, and am angry that the need to spay pregnant cats even exists. Many are not willing to provide that service. And it **is** a service, much as I hate it. People who allow repeated breeding of cats and dogs are to blame, not those trying to prevent it, and certainly not those left to figure out how to fund caring for the unwanted litters.

There are people who, through no fault of their own, have dozens of cats living on their property. Once a few show up and you feed them, more will come. If you try to do the right thing by having them spayed and neutered and ask the vet for a volume discount, they may shame you and call you a hoarder. After that you probably just feel lost.

IHA helps these people. Services are affordable, very high quality, and we specialize in those insane cats you can only capture after many attempts with a humane trap. With our help, farms, trailer-parks and neighborhoods are able be responsible without financial struggle.

So far, despite the number of animals we have sterilized, local shelters are still getting full at puppy and kitten season. Euthanasia at the open-intake shelters still occurs. However, we are lessening that. If the self-righteous can come forward with the space, funds, and manpower, step right up! I will happily be put out of business and play with kittens all day!

Acknowledgements

If I try to list everyone I am thankful to I will miss someone, feel very guilty, and then never be able to look that person in the eye again. But I'll try.

Thank you Carol Woodford, Anya Doll, Chris and Kat Schoon, and Davita Doll-Schmitz, for reading rough drafts that I thought sucked. Thank you, Trish Wasek, for taking a fine-tooth comb for one last edit before mine.

Thank you Cheryl Miller for being the go-between for me and Temple Grandin; and to Temple, for the wonderful words and inspiration.

Thanks to Chris Schoon for reading this and giving a ridiculously kind review.

Thank you Dad and Mom, Jim and Berni Doll, and my siblings Mike Doll, Bill Doll, Marie Doll (God rest her Soul.), Andria Doll, Christi Becker, and Mark Willenbring. You all put up with my "animal phase" as a kid. Gee what happened with that?

Thank you Al, for keeping me as sane as possible throughout college, vet school, and early practice. You put up with the worst of me.

I thank my best friends, Kat Schoon, Chris Schoon, Karla Sibert, John McLaughlin, Trish Wasek, Stacy Dykema, Nicki Brodersen, Jen Read, Steph Oleson, Mary Mincey, Chris McGinnis, and Amy Sacs for tolerating my many annoying habits.

Thank you Joseph Klingelhutz, my son. Thank God you were born will common sense that came entirely from your father. You are wonderful.

Thank you Kris (Kirsten) Platt, my divine super-star daughter. You still seem to think I'm kinda, sorta, maybe, cool to be around. I think.

And finally, thank you Torben Platt, my husband. You are always more confident of me than I am, and have never discouraged me from trying **any** plan or idea I put in front of you, regardless of how outrageous it ends up being. I love you. You have suffered in your own animal adventures, while supporting me in mine. Now go write your own book!

CPSIA information can be obtained
at www.ICGtesting.com
Printed in the USA
LVOW10s1837220318
570824LV00013B/179/P